The Physically Fit Messiah

Wellness Wisdom PAST and PRESENT

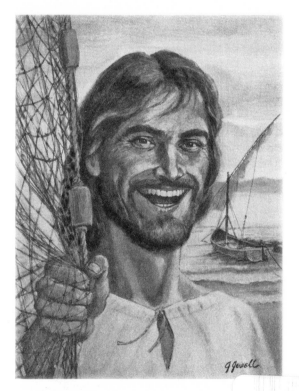

Cal Samra

Robert D. Reed Publishers

Robert D. Reed Publishers
P.O. Box 1992
Bandon, OR 97411
Phone: 541-347-9882; Fax: -9883
E-mail: 4bobreed@msn.com
Web site: www.rdrpublishers.com

This book is published by Robert D. Reed Publishers in cooperation with
The Joyful Noiseletter, P.O. Box 895, Portage, MI 49081-0895
www.joyfulnoiseletter.com

Soft cover ISBN: 978-1-934759-99-8
10-Digit ISBN: 1-934759-99-6

Library of Congress Control Number: 2015957551

Cover Designer and Editor: Cleone Reed
Typist for Author: Robyn Lane
Interior Design and eBook formatting: Susan Leonard
Author photo by Madeline Samra
Cartoons by Jonny Hawkins, Scott Masear, Ron Morgan, Tim Oliphant,
Harley Schwadron, Goddard Sherman, and Ed Sullivan

COVER ART: "The Risen Christ by the Sea" by Jack Jewell.
Copyright © by *The Joyful Noiseletter*.

This book reports on a variety of views of health professionals, nutritionists, and health reformers. The author and publisher do not offer medical
advice or prescribe any form of treatment for ailments without the
approval of a health professional.

Manufactured, typeset, and printed in the United States of America

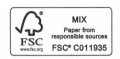

To my sons
Paul, Matthew, and Luke Samra
my granddaughters,
Madeline, Kate, and Lizzie Samra
and the subscribers
to *The Joyful Noiseletter*,
who have filled my life
with healing laughter

Author's Note

In 1986, HarperCollins published my book, *The Joyful Christ: The Healing Power of Humor.* This book is a follow-up to that book, which presented Jesus as a joyful spirit with a keen sense of humor who used humor, as well as prayer, in his healing ministry. He was not the sad-sack Messiah portrayed in many old icons and contemporary Christian paintings. He kept exhorting his followers to "Be of good cheer!"

Jesus attracted children, old folks, and the sick to him—who are not ordinarily attracted to depressives. Amazingly, at the Last Supper, knowing that he is about to be scourged, whipped, tormented, humiliated, and crucified, Jesus is still talking about joy. He tells his disciples: "I have told you this so that my own joy may be in you and your joy may be complete." John 15:11

Down through the centuries, many—though not all—religious figures saw this image of the joyful Christ, including St. Francis of Assisi, Martin Luther, John Wesley, Harriet Beecher Stowe, and G.K. Chesterton.

In 1990, Jack Jewell, a seascape artist, captured the image of a joyful, loving, resurrected Christ in a painting titled "The Risen Christ by the Sea," which graces the cover of this book. The painting was done at the suggestion of Jewell's friend, a chaplain in the New York Fire Department.

The painting, also called "The Easter Laugh," has become extremely popular among Protestants of all faith traditions and Catholics; and *The Joyful Noiseletter*, our newsletter, has distributed tens of thousands of full-color prints of the painting in various sizes. These prints may be ordered from our website—www.joyfulnoiseletter.com—or by calling toll-free 1-800-877-2757.

The painting became the trademark of *The Joyful Noiseletter,* a national humor newsletter which we founded 30 years ago at the urging of many pastors who had read my book *The Joyful Christ.* The pastors wanted a regular newsletter that would provide them and church editors with jokes pastors can tell, inspirational humor, and cartoons they could reproduce in their church newsletters and bulletins.

Through the years, legions of pastors, hospital and military chaplains, church secretaries, medical doctors, nurses, counselors, comedians, humorists, clowns, and cartoonists have contributed items to *The Joyful Noiseletter.* (More information on *The Joyful Noiseletter* and its many editorial contributors is available on its website.)

The Joyful Noiseletter began its ministry over 30 years ago with a focus on the healing power of humor. Through the years, it became increasingly clear to *JN* editors, including the medical doctors on our board of consulting editors, that joy also has a physical component. While we have known many courageous believers who suffer from various ailments or handicaps and yet maintain an attitude of good cheer, it became increasingly obvious to us that it's much easier to be joyful when one is in good health.

Some of the enlightened medical doctors on *JN*'s board of consulting editors and other doctors, nurses, hospital and military chaplains, and counselors who were *JN* subscribers wrote marvelous books on the importance of physical fitness and good nutrition, which we carried in our catalog. They also contributed articles to *JN* on living a healthy lifestyle.

Looking back on the last 30 years of *JN* issues, we were astonished at the number of articles that focused on physical fitness, good nutrition, and health.

This book includes many of the materials from their articles that appeared in *JN*. Many of the wellness tips in this book have been passed on by health professionals. We thank all of the contributors not only for their good humor and good cheer, but also for their wisdom on living a healthy lifestyle.

My book, *The Joyful Christ: the Healing Power of Humor*, described how a couple of very funny pastors helped me recover from a serious, chronic illness by reigniting my faith and my sense of humor. But that wasn't the whole story.

My health improved dramatically after I returned to the organic, natural Mediterranean diet my mother had raised me on, a diet very similar to the food that Jesus ate. And it improved dramatically when I stopped smoking and took up playing tennis four times a week.

The Joyful Noiseletter has received awards for excellence from the Associated Church Press, the Catholic Press Association, and the Evangelical Press Association. But *JN* has never accepted advertising, enabling us to go where angels fear to tread and publish articles without fear that commercial or political interests will withdraw their advertising.

In researching the history of health reformers down through the centuries, we discovered that many Christians of all denominations have made important contributions to public health, detailed in Chapter 1. Many Christians are ignorant of their own history in this respect, or choose to ignore it.

But people of other faith traditions and agnostics, like George Bernard Shaw, also have been valued health reformers. There are those who are so locked into their own theology or philosophy that they ignore or refuse to acknowledge the contributions to public health of those who are not otherwise in their school of thought—altogether very human.

This is not a political tract. Though they may be reluctant to credit one another, both conservatives and liberals have made important contributions to public health.

I also want to thank the following cartoonists, whose cartoons from *The Joyful Noiseletter* have been reprinted in this book: Jonny Hawkins, Scott Masear, Ron Morgan, Tim Oliphant, Harley Schwadron, Goddard Sherman, and Ed Sullivan.

My gratitude also goes to Patch Adams, M.D. for his inspirational work on the healing power of humor, and to my publishers,

Bob and Cleone Reed of Robert D. Reed Publishers for their editorial advice, wise counsel, and enthusiasm for this book.

My thanks to Robyn Lane, a religion major at Kalamazoo College, for entering the manuscript on her computer, proofreading, and for organizing and cataloging the more than 400 books on Christian and Jewish joy and humor that *JN* has received over the years.

Thanks, too, to my granddaughter, Madeline Samra, a speech pathology major at Western Michigan University, for proofreading and assisting me in many ways. And my thanks to Janet Dykens of First Fulfillment, Inc. of Kalamazoo for handling all of the orders from *JN's* catalog so courteously and speedily for many years, and for her good humor and encouragement.

I thank God for the mercies and healings through the years. And special thanks to my beloved mother for steering me back to the healthy, organic Mediterranean diet which she raised me on and which Jesus ate.

Blessings, Peace, and Good Cheer,

Cal Samra
Editor and Publisher
The Joyful Noiseletter
Portage, Michigan

Table of Contents

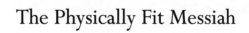

The Physically Fit Messiah

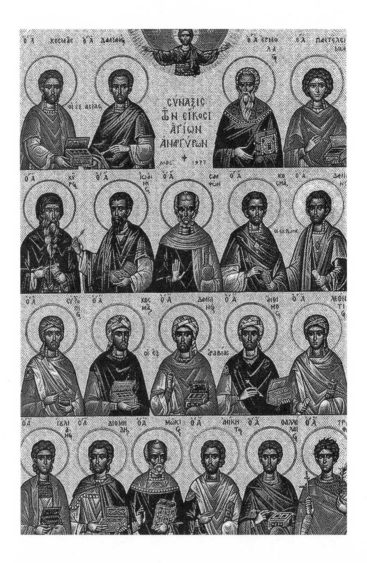

Fr. Michael Taras Miles, pastor of St. Demetrius Ukrainian Catholic Church, Benfield, ND, sent JN this old Greek icon of the 20 "holy unmercenary physicians" from the third century of Byzantine Christianity. They healed people with their prayers, medicinal herbs, nutritious Mediterranean diets, and fasting, and didn't accept money from their patients. They are honored as saints by both the Catholic Church and the Eastern Orthodox Church. St. Cosmas and St. Damian, two Greek brothers, and St. Panteleimon are the best known of them. Some of them were martyred.

Chapter 1

Health Reformers through the Centuries

I went recently to the grand opening in Kalamazoo, Michigan, of Earth Fare, a natural foods supermarket, and was astonished at the huge crowds of young and old people—packed together like sardines—that came throughout the day and week. It was difficult to find a parking space.

Earth Fare calls itself "The Healthy Supermarket" with slogans like "Healthy Food for Everyone," "Love Being Well," "Follow Your Health," and "Items to Keep You Well."

It sells foods that are free of high-fructose corn syrup, bleached or bromated flour, artificial colors, artificial additives and preservatives, and artificial sweeteners. It also sells products and meats that are free from artificial fats and trans fats, antibiotics, and synthetic growth hormones, as well as vegan foods.

Earth Fare partners with farms that grow fruits and vegetables organically, and have a reputation of humane treatment of animals and high-quality meats. "We believe that healthy people grow from healthy bodies, nourished by organic produce," an Earth Fare spokeswoman told me.

Earth Fare, headquartered in Asheville, NC, has expanded into 40 cities in 10 different states.

Trader Joe's, another fast-growing supermarket that specializes in organic and fresh foods and "environmentally friendly stores," now has 418 stores with 85 million visitors throughout America. It's headquartered in Monrovia, California.

(Some of the prices of organic products at these health food stores and markets are higher, but advocates of the natural food movement maintain that the prices will drop as the public demand for these foods increases.)

I've also witnessed the same stampede to purchase healthy fresh produce and the rapid growth of farmers' markets in Kalamazoo, Michigan, and throughout the country with "buy fresh and buy local" slogans. There also has been a widespread movement towards organic gardening and herbal cultivating reminiscent of the Depression gardens of the Great Depression of the 1930's and the Victory Gardens of World War II. Even some hospitals are cultivating organic gardens and buying their foods from farmers' markets.

The number of farmers' markets nationally has increased dramatically from 5,000 in 2008 to 8,000 in 2015.

The millennials—young people in their 20's and 30's and mothers with children—are a leading force in the national natural health food movement, Michael Pollan reports in the fascinating documentary film, "Food, Inc."

Meanwhile, many Americans are flocking to physical fitness clubs.

The Pursuit of Good Health

All this is patently clear evidence that millions of Americans are exercising their constitutional right to pursue not only happiness, but also good health, without which happiness is more elusive.

I wondered why crowds are stampeding to these health-focused grocery stores, farmers' markets, and fitness clubs while church attendance and membership continues to decline in many Protestant, Catholic, and Eastern Orthodox churches. Is it because many churches are blind to the signs of the times and people's hunger for good health? Is it because many churches have neglected Christendom's centuries-old commitment to the health of people? Have they down-played Jesus' reputation as "the Great Physician" who spent many of his days on earth healing people and teaching them healthy life-styles?

Luke was a Greek physician and it is very clear in *Acts* that the Apostles and the early disciples devoted much of their ministry to healing

The Body as a Temple

The Apostle Paul was clearly interested in the health of the body as well as the soul, and in prevention. Paul's admonition in 1 Corinthians 6:19-20: "Do you not know that your body is a temple of the Holy Spirit within you, which you have from God? So glorify God in your body."

Modern Christianity has tended to neglect the health of the body. Few pastors today preach on Paul's admonition. One who does, Rev. Dr. Paul Naumann of St. Michael's Lutheran Church in Portage, Michigan, stresses the importance of "the stewardship of the body."

"Christians are good at honoring the body after you die, but not so much when you're alive," Pastor Naumann observed recently.

Christianity was born as a healing religion, with a special outreach to the poor; and the great appeal of early Christianity was not only that it promised Heaven and the afterlife, but also that it was viewed as a healing faith in this life.

Eat to live; don't live to eat!

–Benjamin Franklin

Many modern clergy as well as the customers who flock to natural food stores, farmers' markets, and physical fitness clubs would be surprised to learn that the pioneers of the modern natural health movement were Christian health reformers from centuries back.

Recapturing Health Ministry

Down through the centuries, various Christian groups in all denominations have striven to recapture the health and healing ministry of Jesus and the early Christians.

These health reformers came from all Christian faith traditions, going back to early Greek Christianity. Among them were Eastern Orthodox Christians, Catholics, and Protestants who disagreed with one another theologically, and may have even ignored the Christian health reformers who came before them.

Today's natural health movement had its beginnings in the Eastern Orthodox and Catholic Churches, to ancient monasteries and monks and nuns who were proficient in organic gardening, herbal treatments, and good nutrition, and who established hospitals to care for the poor.

The First Hospital

The very first hospital was established for the poor and strangers in a Greek community by the saintly monk Basil in the fourth century, and other similar Christian hospitals spread throughout the pagan world.

In the third century, 20 Greek Christian doctors became known as "the unmercenary physicians" because they healed people without charging a fee.

The Merry Franciscans

In the 12th century, St. Francis of Assisi and the early Franciscans were renowned for their healing ministry to the poor. They too healed the sick with prayer, fasting, and medicinal herbs, and by exhorting them to live a healthy lifestyle

The early Franciscans ate a natural Mediterranean diet with lots of fresh fruits and vegetables and whole grains. Like Jesus, the early Franciscans stayed physically fit by walking everywhere. And they sang, laughed, and danced as they went.

(Just about everyone in the Mediterranean countries had—and still has—an organic garden and cultivated medicinal herbs. Numerous modern medical studies have indicated that the Mediterranean diet may well be the world's healthiest diet.)

In the Catholic monastic tradition, the Trappists were vegetarians and esteemed daily physical work.

John Wesley's Health Crusade

In the 18th century John Wesley and the early Methodists became zealous health reformers. When Wesley, the founder of the Methodist movement, realized that doctors in England were available only to the wealthy, he collected health information and published a book, *Primitive Physick*, with practical health tips that pastors and plain people could understand.

Wesley's focus was on prevention. He encouraged pastors to strive to be both spiritually and physically fit, and to instruct church members in a healthy lifestyle.

For Wesley, health was more important than wealth, and the Reformation was ongoing.

He recommended a natural diet close to vegetarian (with modest amounts of animal food) and drinking lots of water. He warned of the dangers to health of cigarette smoking and the intemperate consumption of alcohol. He suggested clergy should get open-air exercise three hours a day by walking or horseback riding. He himself rode endlessly on horseback.

Wesley's book became a bestseller in both England and America.

19th-Century Health Reformers

In the 19th century in America, after the Civil War took a terrible toll in mental and physical ailments, many laywomen, laymen, pastors, and medical doctors from many Protestant denominations spearheaded a widespread health reform movement.

It may come as a surprise to many that the Congregationalist Harriet Beecher Stowe (1811–1896)—famed for her book *Uncle Tom's Cabin*—campaigned just as passionately and wittily for good health, a natural diet, good nutrition and good ventilation in churches, seminaries, medical schools, and trains.

In 1866, this remarkable woman contributed an article to the *Atlantic Monthly* by the intriguing title, "Bodily Religion: a Sermon on Good Health."

Rev. Sylvester Graham, a Presbyterian pastor who invented the Graham Cracker, campaigned relentlessly for a natural plant-based diet, with a focus on fresh vegetables, fruits, and whole grains.

Sojourner Truth was a follower of Sylvester Graham and would take Graham Crackers with her on the trains en route to her speaking engagements.

Ellen White and Dr. Kellogg

Ellen White—another remarkable woman who founded the Seventh-Day Adventist Church—and the Adventists also were a powerful force in focusing on bodily health as a religious duty, extolling the health benefits of vegetarianism, natural foods, and regular exercise.

Another Adventist, Dr. John Harvey Kellogg, a medical doctor and surgeon, also promoted a natural vegetarian diet and regular exercise. Dr. Kellogg founded the famous Battle Creek Sanitarium in Michigan, which attracted thousands of people seeking health and healing for decades.

Dr. Kellogg's sanitarium also extolled hydrotherapy, "the water cure," which sought to heal the sick through the abundant use of fresh water, taken internally or externally through baths and showers.

Dr. Brian C. Wilson, professor of American religious history at Western Michigan University, is an authority on Dr. John Harvey Kellogg and his Battle Creek Sanitarium. In his recent book, *Dr.*

John Harvey Kellogg and the Religion of Biologic Living (Indiana University Press), Dr. Wilson explains Dr. Kellogg's "controversial and uncompromising promotion of vegetarianism:"

> "Dr. Kellogg argued that animal foods putrefied in the body and deposited poisons, thus unnaturally shortening life. Kellogg taught that this was at least in part because animal foods were contaminated with harmful bacteria. Kellogg's nauseating descriptions of the unhygienic nature of slaughterhouses predated those of Upton Sinclair's book *The Jungle* (1906) by several years."

Kellogg, who later had theological disputes with the Adventists, advocated a "religion of biologic living" and had a large following of doctors, pastors, and laypeople from all Christian denominations.

The Adventists, meanwhile, established a network of health food stores near many of their houses of worship.

In the 21st century, the Adventists have gained one million new members every year for the past 10 years, notwithstanding the ongoing theological disputes other Christians have with them. Could this astonishing growth be attributed to the Adventists' relentless focus on bodily health?

(In 1942, the U.S. Army purchased the buildings of Dr. Kellogg's Battle Creek Sanitarium and established the Percy Jones Hospital, which treated some 100,000 World War II military patients.)

Quaker Asylums

In the 19th century, the Quakers established asylums for the mentally ill in Pennsylvania that artfully combined a caring spiritual approach with the best medical care of their times. They were located in restful, idyllic country sites, encouraged their patients to work, and to participate in cultivating organic gardens. They fed their patients a healthful diet of natural foods.

Christian Science

Still another extraordinary woman, Mary Baker Eddy (1821–1910) founded the Christian Science Church in 1879; and by the turn of the 20th century, it had become the fastest growing religion in the United States.

After battling illness as a child and young woman, Mary Baker Eddy was healed through prayer. She wrote a book in 1875 maintaining that sickness is an illusion that can be corrected by prayer alone, that disease is a mental error rather than a physical disorder. No mind, no matter.

To keep the body in good health is a duty; otherwise we shall not be able to keep our mind strong and clear.

–Buddha

She built up a church that would be a return "to primitive Christianity and its lost element of healing."

Christian Scientists testified to many healings through prayer alone. But not all were healed. Christian Science tended to ignore the body, nutrition, physical fitness, and environmental factors, and generally disdained medical and surgical treatments.

In 1907, Mark Twain wrote a satirical diatribe on Christian Science and blistered Mary Baker Eddy as, among other things, "vain, untruthful, arrogant, and illiterate."

Generally, with few exceptions, the Christian health reformers of the 19th century were a humorless lot; and Twain may have been offended that they did not recognize the healing power of humor and a good laugh, which many pastors and doctors appreciate today.

Twain later modified his views of Christian Science when a friend confided to him that he had been healed of neurasthenia after seeing a Christian Science practitioner.

Later, after his daughter, Clara Clemens, became a Christian Scientist, Twain wrote that "the thing behind it is wholly gracious and beautiful."

He also modified his view of Mary Baker Eddy. "In several ways," Twain wrote, "she is the most interesting woman that ever lived, and the most extraordinary."

Christian Science's weakness was in ignoring the God-created body. If your neighbor is poisoning your air, your water, and your food, will prayer alone save you from ill health? And will you be saved by faith or grace alone? That is a question for theologians to contemplate.

Modern Health Reformers

The Christian health reform movement continued into the 20th century. In 1987, Rev. Scott Morris, M.D., a family practice physician and ordained Methodist minister, founded the interfaith Church Health Center in Memphis, TN, to provide quality, affordable health care for working people and their families who are without health insurance.

The Center's focus is on prevention and health education. It has mobilized broad-based financial and volunteer support in the Memphis interfaith community, and cares for over 55,000 patients without relying on government funding.

The Church Health Center is the largest faith-based health care facility in the U.S.

The Church Health Care Center has developed a "Model for Healthy Living" as a tool to help people choose ways to care for their own health. The model urges individuals to take charge of their own health care, and focuses on good nutrition, friends and family, spiritual life, work, regular exercise, cultivating a sense of humor, and medical care.

The Joyful Noiseletter carried a substantial article on the Church Health Center, and also offered in its catalog Dr. Morris' extraordinary book, *God, Health, and Happiness*. In that book, Dr. Morris declared: "Health care is a mess, and churches can help make changes by reclaiming the biblical mandate to bring healing."

The Holistic Nurses

In 1984, Rev. Granger E. Westberg, a Lutheran pastor, hospital chaplain, and teacher of medical students, founded the ecumenical parish nurse movement. Westberg believed that healthcare transcends physical care because true healing involves the whole person.

Westberg wrote a pamphlet titled "How to Start a Church-based Health Clinic." The parish nurse movement grew into Faith Community Nursing with over 16,000 registered nurses, primarily in the United States but also in numerous foreign countries.

The movement integrated the practice of faith with the practice of nursing. Parish nursing is rooted in the Judeo-Christian tradition and the historic practice of professional nursing. But it is not only available to Christian churches. There are also Jewish Congregational Nurses, Muslim Crescent Nurses, and RNs serving within other faith traditions.

Faith Community Nurses serve in several roles, including health advisors, health educators, health screening providers, and visitors of church members at home or in the hospital. Most of them are volunteers, with only about a third of them being compensated for their ministry. They assist members of the faith community to maintain and/or regain wholeness in body, mind, and spirit.

Rev. Westberg's writings also inspired Dr. Scott Morris to found the Church Health Center in Memphis in 1987. The Church Health Center hosts the International Paris Nurse Resource Center Symposium every year in Memphis.

Dr. Russell's "Bible Diet"

JN also featured an article about another contemporary Protestant health reformer, Dr. Rex Russell, and his bestselling book, *What the Bible Says about Healthy Living* (Regal Books), which we also offered in our catalog. Dr. Russell, a *JN* consulting editor, was a radiologist at the Mayo clinic.

He also had a farm in Arkansas. When his health broke down, Dr. Russell, a Baptist, searched the Bible for answers and began to study the physiology of faith. Dr. Russell recovered his health by adding to his diet many of the natural foods which the folks in the Old Testament and New Testament ate, while avoiding the foods that they avoided or ate sparingly. "Your mom was right," Russell wrote, "Eat your fruits and vegetables."

He also recommends doing what those Biblical folks did—an occasional short fast—and exercising regularly.

Patch Adams' Free Hospital

Patch Adams, M.D., "the clown-prince of physicians," also has been a consulting editor to *JN*. The 1998 movie "Patch Adams" told Patch's extraordinary story only in part.

Patch not only is an advocate of the healing power of faith, humor, and love, but he is also hard at work raising funds to realize his dream of establishing the Patch Adams Teaching Center and Clinic in West Virginia.

Patch has enlisted the support of health professionals, including doctors and nurses, who will live and work at the center, along with their patients, and offer free medical services to patients in one of the poorest rural areas in West Virginia.

The clinic's doctors and nurses have committed themselves to work for very modest salaries on 320 acres of land.

The clinic will focus not only on the healing power of humor, play, clowning, and recreation, but also on the health benefits of good nutrition and physical fitness. Both patients and staff will have a hand in creating extensive organic gardens on the land. Patch recommends a balanced, nutritious, plant-based diet, and suggests visitors bring fresh-cut fruits and vegetables on platters for hospital patients and staff.

"My role models of devoted and caring service were Dr. Albert Schweitzer and Dr. Tom Dooley," Patch wrote in his book *Gesundheit!*

"Faith is the cornerstone of our inner strength, a personal and passionate belief in something of inexhaustible power and mystery," Patch told *JN*. "Patients who are full of God need less medication."

Whatever their theological differences, all of these reformers in all centuries had one thing in common: they believed that what goes into your mouth may be as important for your health as what comes out of it.

Lutherans: God's Gardens

In his *Table Talks*, Martin Luther, preoccupied with the serious issues of the Reformation, nonetheless declared: "God is not a God of sadness, but the devil is. Christ is a God of Joy. It is pleasing to the dear God whenever thou rejoicest and laughest from the bottom of thy heart."

Contemporary Lutherans have been at the forefront of the health reform movement. A prominent Lutheran author, Dr. Richard Bimler, president of Wheat Ridge Ministries in Itasca, IL, for many years contributed many articles to *The Joyful Noiseletter* on spiritual and physical health. Dr. Bimler also pioneered health programs for senior citizens.

Wheat Ridge Ministries' mission is "Lutherans seeding new ministries of health and hope in the name of the healing Christ," according to the current president, Richard Herman. "We have been blessed to encourage and assist many reformers through our role as a seeder of new health and human care ministries." Herman said:

"Wheat Ridge Ministries helps health and human care initiatives get off the ground by providing the initial funding and support they need to thrive. Our efforts are focused on improving the health of the whole person by addressing wellness of the body, mind, and spirit. Wheat Ridge Ministries has a special interest in nurturing new health and human care ministries and new faith-based organizations."

Wheat Ridge Ministries gave a grant to St. Stephen's Lutheran Church in Chatham on the south side of Chicago, when the church decided to address the many nutritional problems facing its community, including a limited access to fresh produce and the major health problems resulting from the scarcity of healthy eating options.

Pat Harper, program director of St. Stephen's Healthy Eating/Healthy Living project, said, "We looked around the community and we realized we should have a garden."

The St. Stephen's organic garden just completed its sixth growing season. The 1,200 square-foot garden grows over a dozen different vegetables and fruits, supplying 100 families in the community.

The body is a sacred garment.

– Martha Graham

"We distributed food to those in need," Harper said. "Working the garden gives them training and a positive outlook. It helps turn lives around."

Wheat Ridge Ministries celebrated its 100th anniversary in 2005 by hosting a "National Symposium on Health and Hope in the 21st Century and Beyond" in Denver, Colorado. Over 1,000 health professionals and medical, church, government, corporate leaders, and lay people focused on the theme of "Living Well."

"Living well," said Dr. Bimler, "is taking care of ourselves in body, mind, and spirit so that we can take care of others." There were discussions of diet, nutrition, and environmental factors as they relate to health. Theologian Martin E. Marty was the keynote speaker.

More information on Wheat Ridge Ministries is available on their website: www.wheatridge.org

Of course, not all health reformers are Christian. Many Jews (with their respect for kosher foods), Moslems (with their respect for halal foods—similar to kosher foods), Hindu gurus (with their devotion to yoga exercises and a vegetarian lifestyle), vegetarian Sikhs, and people with no religious beliefs or affiliations have made important contributions to health reform for centuries. Strange bedfellows indeed! It is striking that food has played an important role in the history of all major religions.

One of the most influential health reformers of the twentieth century was an agnostic—the long-lived playwright and humorist George Bernard Shaw. With Shavian Wit, Shaw campaigned relentlessly to educate people to live a healthy lifestyle and to stay physically active. He himself was a confirmed vegetarian.

ObamaCare has been very controversial, but whatever your views of ObamaCare, First Lady Michelle Obama deserves praise for her interest in preventing childhood obesity, her promotion of physical fitness, and her establishment of an organic garden at the White House. Prevention should be a top priority in any health care system, lest the nation goes further into debt subsidizing expensive treatments for diseases that result mainly from unhealthy lifestyles.

Michelle Obama campaigned for a school foods program that set fat, calorie, sugar, grain, and sodium limits on foods in the school lunch line, and urged children to take a fruit or vegetable during lunchtime. She met opposition in some quarters, but said she would "fight to the end" for good nutrition in schools.

We are witnessing a major grass-roots movement led by women and men distressed by the epidemic of obesity and poor health of both children and adults they see as a result of the relentless TV promotion of junk foods, processed foods, and fast foods offered in schools, day care centers, and hospitals.

Healthy Centenarians

An extraordinary recent book, *The Blue Zones: Lessons for Living Longer from the People Who've Lived the Longest* by Dan Buettner, seems to have confirmed the views of Christian and other health reformers down through the centuries.

With the support of *The National Geographic Society*, Buettner led an expedition of medical scientists and health professionals from various disciplines to five areas of the world with some of the world's longest-lived people: communities on Sardinia, Okinawa, Costa Rica, Greece, and Loma Linda, California.

They interviewed many centenarians and discovered that, despite differences in their cultures, they shared certain things in common: they had a cheerful attitude towards life and a sense of humor and laughed a lot; were serious about their faith; had strong, extended-family ties; ate a mainly plant-based diet with a focus on fresh vegetables, fruits, whole grains, beans, nuts, and fish; and stayed physically active. They did not eat fast foods, junk foods, or processed foods full of additives. They did not smoke cigarettes.

A high rate of the seniors in these five communities managed to avoid many of the diseases—like cancer, heart disease, diabetes, depression, Alzheimer's, and dementia—that are crippling and killing many Americans.

In November, 2015, the World Health Organization, based on evidence from hundreds of studies, reported that eating processed meat such as sausages, bacon, ham, cold cuts, and hotdogs causes cancer, placing it in the same category as smoking.

The WHO's cancer research unit classified processed meat, which generally contains pork or beef as "carcinogenic to humans" and linked it specifically to colon, or colorectal cancer.

WHO also defines processed meat as any type of meat that is salted, cured, or smoked to enhance its flavor or preserve it.

WHO also reported that unprocessed red meat such as steak may also be carcinogenic.

It appears that the early Greek physicians, the early Franciscans, the Trappists, John Wesley, Harriet Beecher Stowe, Ellen White, Dr. John Harvey Kellogg, and George Bernard Shaw, among others, were prophetic.

"A preacher is a hospital administrator," Martin Luther said. It also has been said that churches are "hospitals for the sick." If that is so, then why are so many parishioners dying before their time in the pews? If that is so, then why not instruct their congregations on living healthy lifestyles?

Chapter 2

Jesus: The Ultimate Health Reformer and Action Hero

With the widespread public interest in physical fitness, it has somehow been overlooked that Jesus was an amazingly physically fit Messiah. In an age that worships a flock of phony cartoon superheroes, Jesus was the ultimate action superhero 2,000 years ago.

He was a man of great stamina who walked everywhere between the villages of the Holy Land on his ministry of salvation; and there is no record he ever rode a horse, a camel, or a carriage, though he did once enter Jerusalem on a donkey, displaying an ironic sense of humor.

He regularly traveled over hills and climbed mountains. He fished. From time to time Jesus worked as a carpenter, and so was surely lean and muscular, contrasting dramatically with the sedentary clergy of his times. He enjoyed the company of children so much it wouldn't be surprising if he joined them in their games.

He was not a body-builder growing his muscles with weights for show in front of mirrors. Jesus' physical fitness was used in the service of others.

Jesus, the Great Physician, the healer, was supremely healthy, robust, loving, and joyful. Would God have sent us an obese, sickly, depressive Messiah for our salvation? Who would have listened to him? He was a layman. He was the ultimate health reformer.

Jesus, in numerous ways, reminds us again in the Gospels that God made the body to be used in the service of others. Jesus came to us with a message of salvation through both spiritual and physical fitness.

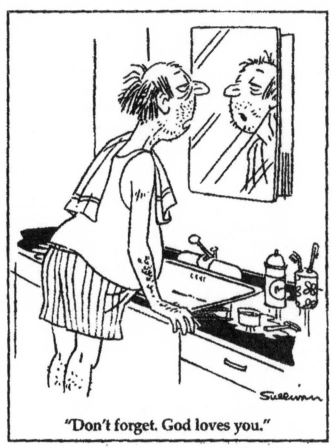

"Don't forget. God loves you."

from *JoyfulNoiseletter.com*
©Ed Sullivan

The Gospels' Action Words

The Gospels, especially Jesus' parables, are replete with action words. The parable of the Good Samaritan is a prime example.

"Faith, by itself, if it has no works, is dead."
(James 2:17)

"But be doers of the word and not hearers only, deceiving yourselves." (James 1:22)

Jesus declared "Not everyone who says 'Lord, Lord,' shall enter the Kingdom of Heaven, but he who does my will." (Matthew 7:21-23)

Jesus reserved his harshest words for those "who say and do not do, for those who preach but do not practice." Jesus called these clergy "lovers of money" (Luke 16:14) and "hypocrites" (Luke 16:14), and, of course, they did not appreciate that.

"Everyone then who hears these words of mine and does them will be like a wise man who built his house upon the rock; and the rain fell, and the floods came, and the winds blew and beat upon that house, but it did not fall, because it had been founded on the rock. And everyone who hears these words and does not do them will be like a foolish man who built his house upon the sand; and the rain fell, and the floods came, and the winds blew and beat against that house, and it fell, and great was the fall of it." (Matthew 7:24-27)

What Did Jesus Eat?

There were no fast-food establishments in Jesus' time, and we know that he was not raised on junk foods and processed foods in day care centers, because there were no day care centers in those days. The Jewish culture of Jesus' time had not experienced the massive exodus from homemaking and child care that modern America has experienced over the past four decades. There were no fast foods restaurants in the Israel of Jesus' time.

We can be certain that his mother, Mary, made a sustained effort to feed her son home cooking and a healthy, natural, Mediterranean diet. It was Mary's labor of love for Jesus, and he was bathed in Mary's love. Jesus was raised on fresh, unprocessed, organic foods free of pesticides, additives, preservatives, food colorings, hormones, et al.

I should rejoice so much that because of joy I remain healthy and cannot become sick. But tiresome Satan works against such joy where he can.

–Martin Luther, *Table Talks*

Like many of the Jewish women of her times, Mary was a masterful nutritionist and cook. Her nutritional knowledge and knowledge of medicinal herbs had been handed down for centuries from mothers to daughters. Mary was not about to raise her Messiah son on junk foods.

Like many people in the Middle East have done for centuries, Mary and Joseph probably maintained an organic garden.

In their book, *The Food and Feasts of Jesus: The Original Mediterranean Diet with Recipes* (Rowan and Littlefield), Douglas Neel and Joel Pugh observe that, in the ancient Jewish culture of Jesus' time, meal preparation was a long process; and peoples' lives revolved around food—from the growing and harvest seasons to the cooking, eating, and storage of the food. The book focuses on everyday meals and the special cuisine prepared for feasts and celebrations.

As observant Jews, Jesus' family did not eat ham or pork. Jesus' meals probably included home-made yogurt, goat cheese, eggs, fish; lots of fresh salads with tomatoes, cucumbers, garlic, and onions, dressed in olive oil and medicinal herbs like oregano, basil, and mint; lots of fresh vegetables like squash, eggplant, and olives; whole-grain wheat, brown rice, lentils, garbanzo beans, nuts like almonds, whole-wheat bread, and honey. He also probably ate an assortment of fresh fruits—figs, dates, apricots, pomegranates, grapes, bananas, apples, and oranges. All these foods are indigenous to the Holy Land.

Very occasionally, for religious holidays and special events, like weddings, Jesus' family probably ate lamb or chicken; but meats were not central to the Mediterranean diet, and, as they are today, meats were used very sparingly in dishes, mainly as seasonings.

Jesus' diet was probably mainly plant-based, and today would come under the category of "health foods" at dear prices. But these health foods were much cheaper in Jesus' time because many families cultivated their own extensive gardens.

Because of the healthy diet Mary fed him and his daily strenuous physical activity, the boy Jesus grew into a strong and healthy man bursting with energy. We also know that Jesus ate in moderation and fasted and prayed frequently, and that he often sought quiet and rest.

Deacon Bob Stevens of St. Monica Catholic Church in Kalamazoo, Michigan, noted that Jesus also occasionally drank some red wine in moderation. After all, he did turn water into wine at a wedding celebration.

The Jews of Jesus' time, including the Apostle Paul, considered wine, drunk in moderation, good for a person; but drunk in excess could be very dangerous, Stevens said.

The New Testament does not specify everything Jesus and his disciples ate at the Last Supper. But any number of Mediterranean fruits and vegetables could have been on the table.

I do not presume to know everything that Jesus ate, or didn't eat. But I'm sure he would have been familiar with, loved, and thrived on, the healthy, organic, Mediterranean cooking of my own Mama. Mama's cooking was probably very similar to Mary's cooking. My mother, whose roots were in the Greek Orthodox Church, could trace her ancestry to the very first Christians of southern Lebanon, which Jesus and his other disciples visited as they sought to convert the Gentiles there. They were the first Christians to be called Christians. (Tragically, many of these Christians whose ancestors were called "the first Christians" 2,000 years ago have fled their homeland because of the endless wars and turmoil of the past century.)

Though she never got past the ninth grade in the French schools of Lebanon, she was a masterful nutritionist, cook, and organic gardener. And when she married my father, she brought her Greek-Lebanese culinary artistry with her to America. She assiduously kept an organic garden in America, just as she had done in Lebanon, and always shopped for fresh fruits and vegetables at farmers' markets. She never read a book on nutrition but she was a nutritional artist.

Our family physician, old Dr. Marshall loved Mama's cooking. Dr. Marshall still made house calls, always arriving with his little black bag, and never charging more than $5 for his services. This was during the latter half of the Great Depression of the 1930s, and Dr. Marshall bartered his services for one of my mother's meals.

Dr. Marshall had come to Michigan after graduating from the McGill University Medical School in Montreal with a specialty in nutrition. As a boy, I remember sitting around the dinner table in our home with Dr. Marshall, who would be ecstatic about the dishes my mother prepared for him.

He especially loved her taboule salad—chopped tomatoes, cucumbers, parsley, onions, lettuce, mint, basil, and whole wheat grain, bathed in an olive oil and lemon dressing.

I remember Dr. Marshall asking my mother what the ingredients were in taboule. And when she told him, he exclaimed, "That's a complete food. If you ate that three times a week, you'd live to a hundred." Mama lived till 96. She also stayed physically active into her old age.

The Poor Woman's Therapy—the Enema

Dr. Marshall believed that a diet that promoted regularity was the key to good health, and Mama's cooking did that.

He was also a believer in enemas, a modification of Dr. John Harvey Kellogg's "hydrotherapy."

When any of our family got sick, Dr. Marshall would tell Mama to make sure that we took an enema. An enema, he said, was a sort of house-cleaning that accomplished what a short fast would do. It was no fun, but we always felt better afterwards.

I remember Dr. Marshall also saying that "American women were the first line of defense against disease." Those were the Depression days, a time when most families could not afford to eat out at restaurants, and when most American women were masterful nutritionists and cooks and insisted on fresh produce.

It was a time when it was considered unethical for doctors, lawyers, and pharmaceutical companies to advertise directly to the public.

"Crunchy Moms" Seek Healthy Lifestyle

I thought of my beloved mother when a pastor called my attention to an extraordinary new organization of independent-minded women who call themselves "Crunchy Moms."

The "Crunchy Moms" web site describes them as follows:

"A Crunchy Mom is a woman on a quest for more information, a Mom who is environmentally, health, and socially conscious. She cares enough about her family to question the status quo.

"She tries to discover the root cause of the problems she observes. When we know better, we do better. A Crunchy Mom is a Mom who fosters a strong, positive bond with her children through natural healthy living.

"A Crunchy Mom sees herself on a journey to find out how best to care for her family in light of both tradition and research."

One of the articles on their website is titled "The Fast Food Monster;" another is "Save Money on Healthy Groceries without Coupons." You can see these articles and join the growing Crunchy Moms community by registering online at crunchymoms.com.

The "Crunchy Moms" seem to be hearkening back to the wise ways of their grandmothers.

How Do You Hang Yourself from a Cactus?

Please forgive this diversion, but we'll return to my Mama's cooking shortly.

In 1986, HarperCollins published my book, *The Joyful Christ: the Healing Power of Humor*, which gave birth to *The Joyful Noiseletter*. That book began as follows:

One sunny morning, I was in the depths of depression and despair, burned out at the tender age of fifty. Everything that could go wrong had gone wrong in my life. My health had greatly deteriorated, forcing me to resign my job in Michigan as a newspaper reporter. My doctor advised me to go to the warmer climate of Arizona, two thousand miles away from my family and friends. I was jobless, looked like skin and bones, and in great emotional and physical pain. I was full of bitterness, anger, self-hatred, fear, and doubt. An urge to be finished with the pain overwhelmed me one day.

I went to a hardware store, bought some sturdy clothesline rope, and drove all over Phoenix and the surrounding desert looking for a suitable tree from which to hang myself. But the Phoenix area has very few trees, and what trees they have are unsuitable for hanging. The palm trees are much too tall to climb, and most everything else is excruciatingly prickly cactus.

I finally drove into the desert near the elegant town of Carefree, sat in the sun next to a very tall cactus, and for a couple hours tried to figure out how to hang myself from it. How do you hang yourself from a cactus?

Finally, I decided that it was all very ridiculous, and that there was no way it could be done—not from a cactus. So I drove around looking for a river to jump into. But all of Arizona's rivers were dry that time of year, with not a drop of water in them.

Then I drove over to Scottsdale and stopped off at La Casa de Paz y Bien, the Franciscan Renewal Center. Something drew me into the chapel, where I found myself down on my knees, praying for the strength to endure my pain and to go on in spite of it.

I have dim memories of that day. But I remember Franciscan Father Gavin Griffith, a warm-hearted Irish wit who could have made a living as a stand-up comedian had he chosen to do so, inviting me to share a meal with him at the center. At dinner, Griffith had me laughing again with his pithy remarks and jokes.

I decided to take a few days' retreat at the center and had the good fortune of getting as a spiritual advisor Franciscan Father Lambert Fremdling, a small, gentle friar who had lived and worked for forty years on an Indian reservation in Arizona. He was a good-humored, elderly man who was a great believer in the siesta.

When the retreat was just about over, Fr. Lambert told me he had something he wanted to give me, and he went scurrying to his office. Soon he returned and gave me a painting of a smiling Christ carrying the imprint "Christ, the Essence of Life, Light, Love, and Laughter."

He said it had been painted by one of his friends, and he wanted me to have it.

The painting gave me a different perspective on Jesus and cast him in a new light.

I was not a Catholic, but the effervescent and good-humored friars and sisters at the Franciscan Renewal Center showed me how to reach out again to other people, to love again, and to laugh again. They rekindled my faith and my sense of humor.

Another priest who befriended me at the Franciscan Center was the jovial Fr. Tom Walsh, who taught a course there titled, "Humor, Hilarity, Healing, and Happy Hypothalami." The famous humorist Erma Bombeck and Fr. Tom had known each other for years at St. Thomas the Apostle Church in Phoenix. Fr. Tom once wrote to Bombeck and asked her whether humor is healing. Bombeck replied with a delightful letter, which she gave me permission to reprint as a prologue to my book. Here it is, in part:

Dear Father Tom:

I suspect you have me confused with Norman Cousins. He's several inches taller, and he laughed his way through illnesses. He got a best-seller out of his illness. I got three children. Those are the breaks.

I am a great believer in your premise that humor heals. I have nothing to back it up physically, but emotionally I have file drawers full of pure testimonials.

I've had pitiful letters from people who swear they don't have a sense of humor and want to know how to develop one, because they've heard how much of a stabilizer one is. And they're right.

I miss you a lot at St. Thomas. Was it something I said?

Erma Bombeck

I also joined a prayer group with both Catholics and Protestants of several faith traditions, and learned to pray for healing not only for myself, but for other people. That strengthened me enormously, as did regular communion, in my journey back to good health.

But there is more to the story of my recovery that did not appear in my book *The Joyful Christ.*

If I can stop one heart from breaking, I shall not live in vain.

–Emily Dickinson, *Apple Seeds*

I had arrived in Phoenix a very sick, beaten, and despairing man. I was in a state of deep depression, had endless gastrointestinal problems and nausea, my weight had dwindled down to 105 pounds, and I could barely walk a half block.

I had tried a variety of remedies popular in my time: psychoanalysis, secular psychotherapies, antidepressants, tranquilizers, but my condition had simply worsened.

My new Franciscan friends had taught me not only the wisdom of Proverbs 17:22—"A cheerful heart is a good medicine, but a downcast spirit dries up the bones."—but also helped me to understand that for years I had been living an unhealthy lifestyle.

Back to the Jesus Diet

As a newspaper reporter in Michigan and New Jersey, I had smoked two packs of cigarettes a day, lived on junk foods, processed foods, TV dinners, fast-foods, hamburgers, French fries, candy, and soda pop.

I'm a slow learner, and it finally dawned on me that when I was living at home and eating my mother's Mediterranean cooking, I rarely was ill but was always strong, healthy, and energetic.

So in Arizona I made a decision to stop smoking and to return to the Mediterranean diet my mother had raised me on—a diet very similar to the diet Jesus ate.

In Phoenix, I also returned to playing tennis almost daily; and the sun, fresh air, and exercise did wonders for my health.

Within six months, I became physically fit, regained my normal weight, and was bursting with energy that I had not experienced before.

I thank God every day for His mercies and for the many instruments of healing He uses: clergy of all faith traditions, friars and nuns, medical doctors, nurses, charismatic laymen and women, musicians, singers, clowns, comedians, and humorists.

Chapter 3

The Healthy Centenarians

*N*ational Geographic recently published an extraordinary book titled *The Blue Zones: Lessons for Living Longer from the People Who've Lived the Longest* by Dan Buettner. This book, which became a bestseller, should be in every church, house of worship, and seminary library in the nation.

With the support of *The National Geographic Society*, Buettner led an expedition of medical scientists and health professionals from various disciplines to four areas of the world with some of the world's longest-lived people, which they called "The Blue Zones."

They interviewed many centenarians and studied their lifestyles, diet, and physical activity in the Barbagia region of Sardinia, an island in the Mediterranean; Okinawa, an island of Japan; the Seventh-day Adventist community in Loma Linda, California; and the Nicoya Peninsula in Costa Rica.

An ounce of practice is worth more than tons of preaching.

–Mahatma Gandhi

A high rate of these longest-living people managed to avoid many of the diseases—like cancer, heart disease, diabetes, Alzheimer's , and dementia—that are crippling and killing many Americans.

The medical researchers discovered that, despite differences in their cultures, the people in these four "Blue Zones" shared certain lifestyles, attitudes, and practices that contributed to their health and longevity.

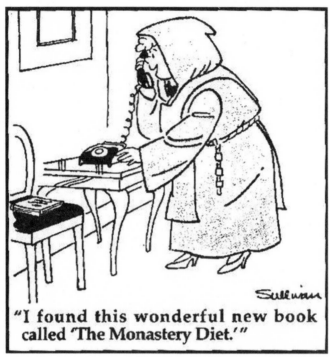

"I found this wonderful new book called 'The Monastery Diet.'"

from *JoyfulNoiseletter.com*
©Ed Sullivan

The centenarians in all four zones retained a cheerful attitude towards life and a sense of humor. Sardinian men shed stress by gathering in the street each afternoon to laugh with and at each other.

The Okinawan women gathered regularly to gossip and crack jokes. One 102-year-old Okinawan woman gave this advice for longevity: "Eat your vegetables, have a positive outlook, be kind to people, and smile."

One elderly Okinawan regularly cycled early in the morning to the beach, swam a half-hour, and then met with a group of other seniors who stood in a circle and laughed. "You smile in the morning and it fortifies you all day long," he said. Buettner observed: "They make it fun and rewarding to be around them."

Of the centenarians interviewed in all four zones, Buettner said, "There's not a grump in the bunch... Studies have shown that a belly laugh a day may keep the doctor away."

The expeditions also found that healthy centenarians everywhere have faith. The Sardinians and Nicoyans of Costa Rica are mostly Catholic. Loma Linda centenarians are Seventh-Day Adventists, a Protestant church founded by Ellen White in the mid-1800s. Okinawans have a "blended religion" that stresses ancestor worship.

Faith and Good Humor

"All belong to strong religious communities. The simple act of worship is one of those subtly powerful habits that seems to improve your chances of having more good years," wrote Buettner.

One Sardinian woman gave a one-word answer on how her mother managed to live so long: "Grandchildren. It's about loving and being loved."

The National Institutes of Health-funded Adventist Health Study found that people who pay attention to their spiritual side have lower rates of cardiovascular disease, depression, stress, and suicide, and their immune systems seem to work better.

"Put generally," Buettner said, "the faithful are healthier and happier."

The centenarians in all four zones were avid gardeners; and their diet was plant-based with a variety of fresh vegetables, fruits, whole grains, beans, nuts, and sweet potatoes.

Sardinians generally ate meat only once a week and for festive occasions, and they drank "artery-scrubbing" red wines daily. Many of the Seventh-Day Adventists were vegetarians; and their faith discourages smoking, alcohol consumption and the consumption of meat.

Yup, gardening and laughing are two of the best things in life you can do to promote good health and a sense of well being.

–David Hobson,
The Mad Gardner

A Japanese physician observed, "The Okinawan culture of longevity was beginning to disappear with the encroaching American fast-food culture," and many of the younger Okinawans are now battling obesity and various ailments.

The centenarians in all four zones had a lean diet and ate in moderation. They got regular, moderate exercise, and walked frequently. They made their hugging, kissing, extended families a priority, and cultivated loving and caring relationships with their families and friends. Their families gave them purpose in life and they honored their elders.

After the book was published, Buettner led another *National Geographic*-funded expedition to study the long-lived inhabitants of the small Greek island of Ikaria.

The Ikarians observe Greek Orthodox Church rituals, have "relentless optimism and a propensity for partying," take daily siestas, walk everywhere, garden, and eat a Mediterranean diet high in whole grains, fresh fruits and vegetables, olive oil, honey, and fish.

The researchers were astonished to find that among Ikarians over 90, there was virtually no Alzheimer's disease or other dementia, conditions which afflict more than 40% of Americans over 90.

U.S.A. *Was* a Blue Zone

Buettner and his scientific team missed one important angle in their book. Had they been able to travel back in time in a time-machine, they would have discovered that much of the United States was a "Blue Zone" in the mid-18th century.

When John Wesley, the founder of the Methodist Church, came to America from England in the mid-18th century, he marveled at the good health of Americans and attributed it to "their continual exercise, universal temperance, moderation in eating, and a natural plant-based diet close to vegetarian."

Ben Franklin made the same observation in his *Poor Richard's Almanac*.

John Wesley, Harriet Beecher Stowe, and Ellen White were right: churches should lead the way in health education. That's what Jesus, "the Great Physician" did.

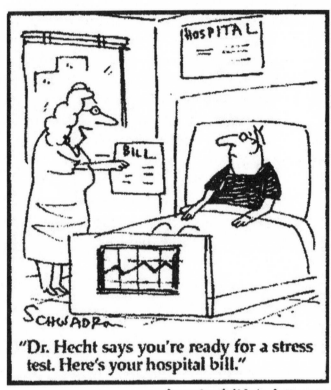

"Dr. Hecht says you're ready for a stress test. Here's your hospital bill."

from *JoyfulNoiseletter.com*
© Harley L. Schwadron

Chapter 4

God Made the Body to Be Used—So Use It!

For centuries, Christian pastors preached on "the seven deadly sins—wrath, greed, pride, lust, envy, gluttony, and sloth." The seven deadly sins were also known as "cardinal sins," and each of them was regarded as a form of "idolatry of the self" and damaging to one's health as well as one's soul.

Pastors used the seven deadly sins to instruct the faithful to avoid them and live a healthy lifestyle.

Two of the seven deadly sins were considered especially damaging to one's health: "gluttony" (overindulgence or over-consumption) and "sloth" (physical laziness or physical inactivity.)

After serving as president of Western Michigan University, Diether Haenicke wrote recently, "The medieval list of deadly sins retains its relevance... and they are plaguing our souls as hard as those of our medieval ancestors."

They are also plaguing our bodies.

In an age of widespread obesity, when was the last time you heard a pastor preach on "gluttony" or "sloth?"

The early Christians looked on physical work as holy—especially physical work on behalf of others. The Apostle Paul earned his living as a tentmaker. In the early Eastern Christian church, many priests in small parishes also had physical jobs.

Probably the early Christians also regarded physical play as holy.

In the 18th century, John Wesley (1703–91), the founder of the Methodist movement, authored a book, *Primitive Physick*, encouraging pastors to strive to be both spiritually and physically fit, and to instruct their church members in a healthy lifestyle.

When Wesley came to America from England, he marveled at the good health of Americans and attributed it to "their continual exercise, universal temperance, and a natural diet."

The Healing Power of Exercise

"In America," he wrote, "diseases are exceedingly few, nor do they often occur, by reason of their continual exercise, and universal temperance."

He suggested that clergy should get open-air exercise three hours a day by walking or horseback riding. Wesley estimated that he himself rode on horseback 250,000 miles in his long lifetime.

My great-grandfather was a Greek Orthodox priest in Lebanon during the early part of the 20th century. (Orthodox priests can marry if they do so before they are ordained.) He was a horseback rider all of his life and was even riding horseback well into his nineties, traveling between the mountain villages of southern Lebanon.

He was a highly respected peacemaker, who was often asked to mediate disputes between the Orthodox, Greek Catholic, Maronite Catholic, Druze, Shiite Moslem, and Sunni Moslem villages.

A loving, gentle, and brave man, he lived to the age of 98. (I suspect his longevity was also helped by the natural, organic, Mediterranean diet he ate.)

My great-grandfather was a kindred spirit to John Wesley, another relentless horseback rider.

In his book, *Primitive Physick*, Wesley wrote, "The power of exercise, both to preserve and restore health, is greater than can well be conceived; especially in those who add temperance thereto... and steadily observe both that kind and measure of good habits which experience shows to be most friendly to health and strength."

Some of Wesley's exercise suggestions might be considered laughable today. Wesley suggested, "Those who read or write much should learn to do it standing; otherwise it will impair your health."

That might be incredible advice in an age of office workers sitting at computers for hours.

But hold on! Wesley was prophetic. British experts recently recommended that office workers stand for at least two hours a day, the Associated Press reported.

In an article published by the *British Journal of Sports Medicine*, the experts of Public Health England warned against the dangers to the health of prolonged sitting.

Bradley Gavin, director of a group called Get Britain Standing, compared the hazards of sitting too much to those of smoking, with research finding that people who spend most of their days seated are more likely to be fat, have heart problems, and cancer, and even die earlier.

The British experts recommend that people start with two hours of standing, and eventually double that to four hours.

Bradley noted that 95% of adults in developed countries are classified as inactive, and that curbing the amount of time people spend sitting can have huge health benefits.

Exercise Dissipates Depression

Exercise also helps dissipate depression. One of *The Joyful Noiseletter's* consulting editors, Donald L. Cooper, M.D., is an authority on sports medicine and physical fitness. He's a nationally recognized physician honored by President Reagan.

Dr. Cooper has impressive medical credentials. He was appointed to the President's Council on Physical Fitness and Sports by President Reagan in 1981. He was football team physician and director of the Student Health Center at Oklahoma State University in Stillwater, Oklahoma. He was the U.S. Olympic Team Physician in Mexico City in 1968.

You'd be surprised, then, to learn that Dr. Cooper fought a couple of heroic battles with depression that crippled him, hospitalized him, and brought him to the edge of suicide.

Dr. Cooper, a devout Presbyterian, attacked his depressive episodes with faith, prayer, exercise, and a sense of humor.

When depression first struck him in 1958, Dr. Cooper was living the American Dream. He had a wife, three children, a new home, and a busy general practice. For no apparent reason, he began waking repeatedly at night, panic-stricken, his mind racing. He began experiencing feelings of failure, hopelessness, and despair. He even began considering suicide.

"The pain of depression is ever so much worse than physical pain," he said. "I have experienced both. Physical pain is so much easier to deal with. Psychic pain is there 24 hours a day, all-consuming. It gets you from the top of your head to the end of your toes, and everything in-between hurts. A person is willing to do anything to get away from it."

Cooper signed himself into the VA Hospital in Topeka, Kansas. "I was an extremely angry young man," he recalls. "I'd beat on the punching bag for a couple of hours every day."

Cooper recovered after three months, and returned to a normal life. In 1979, he suffered from another depression, but again rode it out with professional help, medication, and the love and support of his family.

Dr. Cooper has these suggestions for a person suffering from depression:

> "Keep talking to doctors, counselors, pastors, and friends until you find the right person to talk to.

> "Never medicate yourself. Let the professionals prescribe the medication.

> "Exercise. Movement is medicine.

> "The more fresh fruits and vegetables you eat, the better off you are.

"Cultivate a sense of humor. ("I give 30 to 40 lectures a year on stress management," he says, "and my No. 1 emphasis on managing stress is laughter.") (He became a popular speaker and peppered his lectures with humor and jokes.)

"Hang on to your faith."

Teddy Roosevelt also beat depression by horseback riding and not looking back.

As a child and as a young man, Theodore Roosevelt suffered from asthma and bouts with depression. His depression deepened after both his young wife and his mother died from illnesses on the same night.

His father, a devout Christian, advised him to keep the faith, go west, build up his body with lots of exercise, and help others less well-to-do than he was. Roosevelt went to South Dakota and became a cowboy.

"Black care rarely sits behind a rider whose pace is fast enough," Roosevelt said.

His depressions dissipated, and Roosevelt returned to become one of America's wittiest and most energetic presidents, however controversial.

Roosevelt also became one of the nation's greatest conservationists, environmentalists, and health reformers. He promoted good nutrition.

In 1906, Upton Sinclair created a public uproar with his best-selling, muckraking novel, *The Jungle*, which exposed deplorable conditions in the U.S. meat-packing industry and aroused the public to marketplace hazards.

Sinclair's close friend was a Christian pastor, Rev. William Moir, though he himself was a critic of Christianity. President Teddy Roosevelt thought that Sinclair was a bit kooky, but he agreed with Sinclair that "radical action must be taken to do away with the efforts of arrogant and selfish greed."

The public uproar led to Roosevelt's 1906 Pure Food and Drug Act and the Meat Inspection Act, which prohibited the interstate transport of goods that had been "adulterated;" and Roosevelt pursued an aggressive campaign against manufacturers of food with chemical additives.

The Beginning of the FDA

Roosevelt's campaign also led to the establishment of the Food and Drug Administration, which is responsible for protecting and promoting public health through the regulation and supervision of food safety, animal foods and feeds, dietary supplements, tobacco products, prescription drugs, et al.

In 1917, a retired Roosevelt wrote:

> "In this world, a churchless community—a community where men have abandoned and scoffed at or ignored their religious needs is a community on the rapid down-grade.
>
> "I advocate a man's joining in church works for the sake of showing his faith by his works. The man who does not in some way connect himself with some active, working church, misses many opportunities for helping his neighbors, and therefore, incidentally, for helping himself."

"My First 100 years"

In 2007, *The Joyful Noiseletter* carried a story about the amazing Waldo McBurney (October 3, 1902—July 8, 2009) who at age 104 had just written a book titled *My First 100 Years! A Look Back from the Finish Line*.

McBurney, who was still serving as an elder at the Reformed Presbyterian Church in Quinter, Kansas, had been working at a variety of physical jobs since the age of 13, and had never stopped working.

At the age of 65, he took up long-distance racing, the long jump, and shot put in the Senior Olympics, and set records into his 90's. At the age of 91, he became a beekeeper and sold honey from his office.

"I don't think retirement is in the Bible," McBurney says. "The Bible says God will supply all your needs."

McBurney attributed his longevity to his balanced life, including a strong faith, a sense of humor, a healthy natural diet, a lifestyle full of physical activity, and rest. A lifelong gardener, he grew and ate over 30 different fruits, vegetables, and herbs—"fresh out of the garden without shelf-life deterioration, or possible pesticide pollutants." He also favored whole grains.

His book's back cover proclaimed: "A merry heart is a good medicine." (Proverbs 17:22) McBurney's other favorite bits of wisdom: "Motion is the best lotion." "My food is my medicine and my medicine is my food." "The Lord is my strength." (Exodus 15:2)

"Conducting Can Improve Your Health"

Some people believe they can face aches, pains, depression, tension, or anger only with the help of pills and drugs. Medication can help, but Dr. Dale L. Anderson also believes in stimulating the divinely created "internal pharmacy" in your head.

The Minnesota physician touts the body's production of endorphins, chemicals he calls "inner uppers" that help make us healthy and "high on life." Dr. Anderson believes that laughter is among the best ways to produce these pharmaceutical marvels, along with faith, exercise, singing, and positive mental images.

To get the body to release endorphins, Dr. Anderson has invented an enjoyable method he calls "J'ARMing"—jogging with the arms. He has demonstrated this physical activity, which resembles conducting an orchestra with the wave of a baton, to thousands of patients and workshop participants. Persons who "J'ARM" can use chopsticks, forks, pencils, or other assorted objects to conduct. He says:

"J'ARMing" improves the flow of blood to the brain, produces more endorphins, and strengthens immune systems... Laughter truly is the best medicine. The good feelings which we Christians get from prayer, belief, hope, love, joy, etc. are undoubtedly the result of divinely created chemicals which these positive feelings produce in our bodies. Religion and following Christian teachings are ways to raise these beneficial chemicals."

He has produced a book and a cassette about "J'ARMing." His wife calls him Prince "J'ARMing."

Once a successful surgeon, Dr. Anderson had to give up surgery because childhood burn injuries to his hands eventually prevented his wearing surgical gloves, Now 82, he travels the world touting the benefits of health education via "J'ARMing."

For his patients and audiences, the doctor often orders a "fake laughter prescription" consisting of standing before a mirror for 15 seconds twice a day and enjoying a hearty belly laugh.

Dr. Anderson suggests that persons everywhere should "attack life with silliness." He makes sure that people attending his seminars sing silly songs with him. "I'm not offering a panacea," Dr. Anderson says, "but health education should be a lot more exciting than it has been. It should be health entertainment."

Dr. Anderson is a member of the United Church of Christ in Falcon Heights, Minnesota.

His Dad Walked His Way to a Long Life

In a delightful tribute to his father, Michael Gartner, former president of NBC News, reported that his father quit driving in 1927, when he was 25 years old, and walked everywhere or took streetcars or buses for 77 years. "I decided," he told his son," that you could walk through life and enjoy it or drive through life and miss it."

Gartner's mother was a devout Catholic, and his father an "equally devout agnostic." Nearly every morning for 20 years, he would walk with her the mile to the Catholic church for Mass.

She would sit in the front pew, and he would wait in the back until he saw which of the parish's two priests was celebrating Mass that morning.

"If it was the pastor," Gartner recalled, "he'd take a two-mile walk, meeting my mother at the end of the service and walking her home. If it was the assistant pastor, he'd take just a one-mile walk and then head back to church to meet my mother. He called the two priests 'Father Fast' and 'Father Slow.'" He had a terrific sense of humor.

Gartner's mother finally learned to drive in 1952 when she was 43, and she drove the family car until she was 90, accompanied by his father. But they walked together often. Gartner's father continued to walk daily, and when he was 101, he had his son get him a treadmill because he was afraid he'd fall on the icy sidewalks, but he wanted to keep exercising. He was of sound mind and sound body until the moment he died at age 102. Gartner wrote:

> "I miss him a lot, and think about him a lot. I've wondered now and then how it was that my family and I were so lucky that he lived so long. I can't figure out if it was because he walked through life.
> "So love the people who treat you right.
> "Forget about the ones that don't."

A 600-Mile Walk

JN subscriber Edward R. Sunshine, a former professor of theology at Barry University, and his daughter Ellen recently completed a 600-mile walking tour with 23-pound backpacks across the northern part of Spain—from the snow-packed Pyrenees mountains, down valleys, up treacherous ridges, and over plateaus to the coast, Sunshine described the walk as a very physical and spiritual experience.

"Joggling" Kept Pastor Fit and High-Spirited

"Joggling" helped keep Pastor Mike Hout physically fit as well as spiritually fit.

After he was ordained, Hout discovered that he was putting on a lot of weight because he was mostly sitting around talking to people and reading and writing sermons. Hout, pastor of Good Shepherd Lutheran Church in Kettering, Ohio, decided to trim down by taking up "joggling"—juggling while running.

Hout made the 1994–1995 *Guinness Book of World Records* for setting a world record of 20 seconds in the 110-meter hurdles while juggling three balls. He taught juggling to his wife, Cindy, and their three teenage sons; and the Hout family collected five individual medals at the 46th International Juggling Association Festival. Hout also started a juggling group at his church, and gave free juggling classes to poor people in the Dayton inner city while sharing the Gospel.

"Sophiea!" ("Wisdom" in Greek)

Father Stylianos Muksuris, who has served several Greek Orthodox churches in the United States since emigrating from Greece, has a cell phone programmed to play "Beethoven's Ode to Joy" whenever someone calls him. Even if the voice on the other end is whining or complaining, the music reminds the priest that the eternal God remains a God of peace and joy.

Muksuris is also a powerful advocate for physical fitness. In 1998, he tipped the scale at over 260 pounds, and his blood pressure readings shot upwards. He became concerned that his love for rich, processed foods and sugars and his sedentary lifestyle were damaging his health.

He cut out junk foods and soda pop, and ate lighter, balanced meals with cereals, salads, and fruits. He also began walking three miles a day.

His weight-loss program was difficult at first, he said, but "I always kept it in my mind that I was doing it for my wife and young daughter, and to be better able to serve the members of my parish."

He also developed a greater appreciation for the Orthodox Church's numerous fast and food-abstinence days. For instance, Orthodox believers are asked to avoid all meat and animal products during the Advent and Lenten periods.

It was slow-going, but in a year-and-a-half, Fr. Muksuris lost 60 pounds; and his blood pressure dropped down to a normal 120/70. He also felt better and gained energy.

"As I lost weight," Fr. Muksuris said, "my mood also improved. When I was heavier, I used to be more irritable. Things would bother me then that don't bother me now. I discovered that the body affects the mind, and the mind affects the body."

Fr. Muksuris' story was told in both *Prevention* magazine and *The Joyful Noiseletter.* He later became a bishop in the New York office of the Greek Orthodox Church in America.

A Very Fit Little Old Lady

Down the block from our house in Portage, Michigan, lived a 91-year-old Greek woman who had immigrated to America three years earlier to live with her son and his family. She was a small, lean woman; and in the summer I would see her walking to the local grocery store with two empty shopping bags, and then walking back with the two bags filled with groceries. She still cooked for her son, daughter-in-law, and grandchildren. The family went to the local Greek Orthodox Church on Sundays.

In the summer I would see her using an old-style, hand-powered lawnmower to mow her lawn. In the winter after a blizzard on a bitterly cold day, I spotted this tiny woman, wearing a long black dress and a modest coat, who obviously weighed less than 100 pounds, diligently shoveling snow with a hand-shovel on the sidewalk in front of her home after her son and grandsons had gone to work.

On both sides of the woman's house, two husky, 250-pound men were huffing and puffing as they both used self-propelled snow blowers to clear the sidewalks in front of their own homes.

I wish I had a camera to capture the scene, a Norman Rockwell painting. These old country women were very feminine but they were tough, I thought; she reminded me of my mother.

Church Opens Fitness Center

It became increasingly difficult for African-American pastor Addis Moore to visit people in the hospital who were suffering from preventable diseases, and to conduct funerals for younger people who had died from treatable conditions such as high blood pressure or diabetes.

Rest is only found in action.

–P.T. Barnum

So Rev. Moore spearheaded a project by his church, Mount Zion Baptist Church in Kalamazoo, Michigan, to open its new $200,000 Living Well Fitness Center near the church.

"We pray for sick people, but we decided we needed to do something else," Moore said. "Our goal is to reach people who don't exercise and eat right."

An Associated Press story from Atlanta described a wellness and weight-loss program called First Place, which started at First Baptist Church in Houston, Texas, and now operates in about 10,000 churches. One woman said: "We memorize a Scripture verse and recite it when we stand on the scales."

Carole Lewis, national director of First Place, explained: "We have people who know Christ, so spiritually they're OK, but they are so out of balance physically and they have no joy. There are a lot of Christians who are extremely overweight."

Pastor David Sidwell of Immanuel Lutheran Church in Kalamazoo, Michigan, made a point in a summer sermon recently to encourage his congregation to take time "for both physical activity and paying attention to fresh foods and healthy cooking." He encouraged church members to take daily walks and patronize the farmers' markets in the area.

"Consider your body as a 'temple of the Lord,' as an encouragement to healthy exercise and healthy eating. This summer could be the beginning of good habits that could continue throughout the year," he said.

The Kings of Exercise

Two of the most famous physical culturists of modern times, Bernarr Macfadden (1868–1955) and Jack LaLanne (1914–2011) did not identify themselves with any religious movement, but both of them stressed the importance of positive thinking in maintaining good health; and they clearly were influenced by the teachings on diet, fasting, and exercise of John Wesley, Ellen White, and Dr. John Harvey Kellogg.

Macfadden, considered "the father of physical culture," was sickly and weak as a young child. As a youngster, he took a job on a farm, and the hard physical work and farm-fresh food transformed him into a physically fit and strong young man. He became a vegetarian and opened vegetarian restaurants that featured raw vegetable diets. He popularized the practice of short fasts. And he campaigned tirelessly against processed foods, bread (which he called "the staff of death,") and health professionals he called "pill-pushers."

Macfadden built up a vast publishing empire, publishing magazines on health and body-building. He also attracted many critics, who included his four wives. He was married four times.

Macfadden also promoted in his magazine, *Physical Culture*, another famous physical culturist, Charles Atlas (1892–1972), who became a popular body builder of the 1930s and 1940s. Atlas (born Angelo Siciliano in Italy) came to New York and prospered with a relentless, iconic advertising campaign about "the 97-pound weakling" who became a strongman with Atlas' system of exercise, mirroring Atlas' own transformation.

Atlas also promoted his own health food stores.

Following in Macfadden's and Atlas' footsteps, Jack LaLanne was an American physical fitness and nutritional expert who was called "the godfather of fitness" in the 1950s and onwards.

As a child, LaLanne described himself as "runty and pimply, a troublemaker and juvenile delinquent with a sour disposition and blinding headaches." As a teenager, he once set his house on fire. He described himself as a "sugarholic" and a "junk food junkie" with behavioral problems until he was 15.

His life was turned around when his mother took him to hear a lecture by a physioculturist-nutritionist who told him to stop eating junk foods and start exercising daily. He changed his lifestyle dramatically, and for the rest of his life ate nothing but raw vegetables and fruits. He started out as a vegetarian but later added fish to his diet. And he exercised two hours a day, seven days a week. He ate ten raw vegetables and several pieces of fresh fruit daily, raisins, and nuts.

"Some people thought I was a nut," LaLanne said, "and some doctors were against me." But LaLanne persevered and got a huge national television audience for "The Jack LaLanne Show" (1953–1985). Children and the elderly joined him in his exercise routines on his television show, while he discussed good nutrition and his dog, "Happy," performed tricks.

LaLanne became famous for his prodigious feats of strength. At age 70, handcuffed, he towed 70 boats carrying 70 people while swimming a mile and a half through Long Beach Harbor.

At age 88, LaLanne was still waging war against a disease he called "flabbyseatitus." "Would you get your dog up in the morning and give it coffee, cigarettes, and doughnuts?"

He often stressed that artificial food additives, drugs, and processed foods contributed to making people mentally and physically ill.

When he went to Philadelphia to promote a healthy lifestyle for overweight Philadelphians, he told Art Carey, a reporter for *The*

Philadelphia Inquirer: "A palooka who stuffs his face with potato chips and lifts only the TV remote may be 45 by the calendar but may have a fitness age of 60. Conversely, a yuppie who rides her bike to work and climbs stairs instead of taking the elevator may be 35 according to her birth certificate but have a fitness age of 22."

"People work at dying," LaLanne said. "They don't work at living. Exercise is the king, and nutrition is the queen."

Other health reformers might have put it differently: "Jesus is the king: exercise, nutrition, and humor are the servants."

15 Exercises to Avoid

1. Jumping on the bandwagon.
2. Wading through paperwork.
3. Running in circles.
4. Pushing your luck.
5. Spinning your wheels.
6. Adding fuel to the fire.
7. Beating your head against the wall.
8. Climbing the walls.
9. Beating your own drum.
10. Dragging your heels.
11. Jumping to conclusions.
12. Grasping at straws.
13. Fishing for compliments.
14. Throwing your weight around.
15. Passing the buck.

—*Apple Seeds*

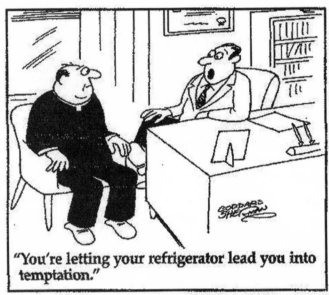

"You're letting your refrigerator lead you into temptation."

from *The Joyful Noiseletter*
© 2000 Goddard Sherman

Chapter 5

Many People Dig Their Graves with Their Teeth

"Many people dig their graves with their teeth," wrote that great humorist George Bernard Shaw, who lived to the ripe old age of 94. Shaw was an agnostic health reformer, a lean promoter of vegetarianism and exercise, who may have had more in common with St. Paul, John Wesley, and Ellen White than he supposed.

Shaw also campaigned against vivisection—surgical and other experiments performed on living animals—and skewered with Shavian wit the Russian scientist Pavlov for his experiments on dogs.

Shaw grieved when his good friend, the great English Catholic humorist G.K. Chesterton, with whom he had a series of splendid public debates, died at the young age of 62. Chesterton's weight had ballooned beyond 300. Chesterton arguably had been Christianity's foremost defender of the 20th century, but he never grasped the physiology of his faith.

The merry-hearted Chesterton is one of my favorite humorists. He famously wrote, "Angels can fly because they take themselves lightly. Never forget that the devil fell by force of gravity."

Chesterton's early demise may be a lesson to all of us that no matter how brilliant we are, the devil is able to find chinks in our armor. And there are things that Christians can learn from agnostics.

I've lived long enough to have known many friends and good men and women—ministers, priests, bishops, doctors, and devout laypeople—who went to their graves because of diseases caused by obesity, poor nutrition, cigarette smoking, and a physically inactive lifestyle. I wept as I watched them battle bravely but succumb to heart disease, diabetes, cancer, tumors, strokes, or Alzheimer's.

Gluttony was taken seriously as one of the seven deadly sins until, ironically, the modern Age of Obesity, when you rarely hear a preacher talk about it, lest he offend the overweight people in his congregation, or call attention to his own hefty weight.

> *Work hard in your flower or vegetable garden and tranquilizers or psychiatrists won't be necessary.*
>
> –Jim Reed

We are in the midst of a world-wide obesity epidemic. Statistics indicate that 30% of Americans are now obese or overweight, and in two decades, 95% of all Americans will be obese or overweight, and many will have diabetes. In two decades it will be difficult to find a passing lane on city sidewalks.

Dr. Robert Lustig, a pediatrician, reports that obesity is an epidemic in babies, children, and adults. One in ten children was overweight in times past; now one in five is overweight.

Obesity kills. Jim Landers reported in *The Dallas Morning News*: "Clogged arteries and sedentary lifestyles have replaced germs as the world's leading killers. Where hunger once held much of the world in its grip, the number of overweight and obese people—1.6 billion—now outnumber those who are malnourished 2 to 1."

You don't have to spend millions in research to observe hospital waiting rooms where extended families gather while a relative is undergoing surgery for various ailments. Typically, both the patient and the extended family are obese or overweight.

You can also see it in all-you-can-eat buffet restaurants, where folks gorge themselves, a prelude to an inevitable trip to a doctor or hospital.

Christopher Ingraham reported in *The Washington Post*: "The growing girth (of both American women and men) basically boils down to three factors: we're eating less healthy food, we're eating more of it, and we're not moving around as much."

A study published in the journal *BMC Public Health* found that Americans are now the world's third-heaviest people. The average American is 33 pounds heavier than the average Frenchman, 40 pounds heavier than the average Japanese citizen, and 70 pounds heavier than the average citizen of Bangladesh.

Numerous medical studies have connected obesity to diabetes, heart disease, cancer, and depression.

The Babe's Bellyache

"The Bambino," "The Sultan of Swat," Babe Ruth (1895–1948) was one of America's greatest and most loveable sports heroes. He set numerous hitting records in his 22-year career, mainly with the New York Yankees.

He endeared himself to the public by often visiting children in orphanages and hospitals, and by signing thousands of autographs without asking a dime for them.

Ruth was lean and muscular in the early years of his career, but he had a voracious appetite and he ballooned to 260 pounds. In 1925, he became seriously ill and was hospitalized with what became known as "the bellyache heard 'round the world."

Sportswriter W.O. McGeehan wrote that Ruth's illness was due to binging on hotdogs and soda pop before a game. His doctors advised him to take better care of himself, stop drinking, womanizing, and gorging himself. They put him on an austere training program, and he recovered to have some of his best years in the majors.

But soon he was back to his old habits, his weight ballooned again, and he was forced to retire in 1935. In 1946, he became ill with cancer, and died in 1948 at the young age of 53. An entire nation mourned. It's mind-boggling to think of the records Ruth would have set had he listened to his doctors and taken care of himself.

Another loveable Major League baseball player, the African-American Gates Brown, was one of the game's all-time greatest pinch-hitters. He helped the Detroit Tigers to the 1968 world championship.

Brown also had a voracious appetite for hotdogs. In 1968, Mayo Smith, the Tiger manager, had a strict rule that players could not eat in the clubhouse during games.

Brown secretly bought two hotdogs from a vendor, stuffed them in his jersey, and sat on the clubhouse bench. He was surprised when the manager called him to pinch-hit early in the game. Brown hit a double and slid head-first into second base. "I had mustard, ketchup, hot dogs, and buns all over me," he recalled. The players in the Tiger dugout and the opposing players all erupted with laughter.

Brown's weight also ballooned throughout the years, and he was in failing health the last years of his life. He died of a heart attack at age 74.

In contrast, here's how a dramatic change in diet helped heal another baseball player:

In 2014, Jose Iglesias, the slick-fielding, 25-year-old shortstop of the Detroit Tigers suffered two shin fractures on both legs and was forced to sit out the rest of the season. His doctors treated him with physical therapy and a major change in his diet, the *Detroit Free Press* reported. He adjusted his diet to include more fresh, green vegetables and broccoli.

Iglesias made a dramatic recovery, returned to play shortstop regularly in 2015, hit over .300, and was named to the All-Star team. His shin fractures were completely healed. He had not been a fan of vegetables, he said, "but I think every time you improve your diet you improve your physical condition."

A remarkable documentary film, *Super Size Me*, was produced and televised in 2004. Directed by and starring Morgan Spurlock, an independent filmmaker, the film follows a 30-day period in 2003 in which Spurlock ate only McDonald's food.

Spurlock dined at McDonald's restaurants three times per day for 30 days, eating every item on the chain's menu. He consumed the equivalent of nine Big Macs per day during his experiment.

As a result, Spurlock, then 32, gained 24 pounds, a cholesterol level of 230, and experienced mood swings, sexual dysfunction, and fat accumulation in his liver.

It took Spurlock, a healthy, physically fit man when he began the experiment, 14 months to lose the weight gained from his experiment. He lost the weight by switching to a vegan diet.

The best place for your bathroom scale is in front of your refrigerator.

–Jim Reed

The film documents the fast-food lifestyle's drastic impact on Spurlock's physical and emotional well-being, and it explores the fast food industry's corporate influences, including how it encourages poor nutrition for its own profit.

The documentary was nominated for an Academy Award for Documentary feature. It is available as a DVD. There is also a paperback book titled *Super Size Me*, published by LENNEX Corp. in Scotland.

A friend of mine joined a Catholic church about the same time a new priest was assigned there. The new priest was rotund, weighing nearly 300 pounds, and was never seen to smile or walk anywhere. He had been trained as a clinical psychologist, and his weekly sermons were full of psychobabble oddly wrapped around a Gospel reading.

He had one relentless passion. He loved a fast-food restaurant near the church. In the morning, he would drive there for breakfast and order eggs, sausage, fries, toast, and coffee. He would drive there for lunch and order two cheeseburgers, fries, and soda pop. And he would drive there for dinner, and have two more cheeseburgers, fries, soda pop, and ice cream. He also smoked.

His girth grew and grew, and sadly he died of a heart attack at the youthful age of 56.

Like some of today's clergy, he had forgotten, or never learned, the time-tested principles of his own faith.

The Apostle Paul valued moderation as benefitting both body and soul. "Let your moderation be known unto all men," he advised the followers of Jesus. (Philippians 4:5)

Paul also warned against drunkenness, but he said in 1 Timothy 23, "No longer drink only water but use a little wine for the sake of your stomach and your frequent ailments."

A *little* wine.

Television daily bombards us all with fast-food and soda pop commercials. One health-minded osteopathic physician recommends to his overweight and obese patients that they simply use their remote control to change channels when a commercial pops up.

It's unnerving when you hear NBC-TV News disclosing an FDA report that 48 million Americans get sick from food-borne illnesses such as salmonella. So what is the FDA doing about all this food-poisoning?

Columnist Al Lewis wrote recently in *The Wall Street Journal:*

> "America is the land of the free, and its citizens live the shortest and sickest lives of anybody in the world's most-developed nations.
>
> "If you want to live past age 50, your odds are better in 16 other developed nations, according to a study by the Institute of Medicine and the National Research Council.
>
> "The study lists cars, drugs, and guns among the leading causes of death for those under 50.
>
> "The solution for every problem in the U.S. is always more. This is why we kill ourselves, trying to get more of everything.
>
> "We are the land of plenty, which means an average intake of 3,770 calories a day, obesity, diabetes, and heart disease, according to the report.

"Anyone who watches TV knows advertisers sell causes and cures in back-to-back commercials.

"Our diseases are mostly the result of our appetites. And advertisers manipulate our appetites at our eyes' every turn.

"You are free to indulge excessively. This keeps the corporate machinery humming."

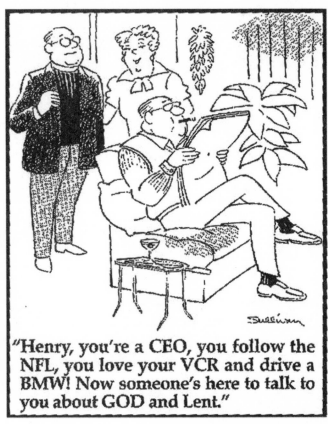

"Henry, you're a CEO, you follow the NFL, you love your VCR and drive a BMW! Now someone's here to talk to you about GOD and Lent."

from *JoyfulNoiseletter.com*
©Ed Sullivan

Chapter 6

Old Greek Lenten Fast Was a Spring Housecleaning

Fr. Michael Taras Miles, pastor of St. Demetrius Ukrainian Catholic Church, Belfield, North Dakota, searched the old Byzantine Christian Lenten liturgies and discovered numerous references to joy.

Joy during Lent? The 40-day "Great Fast" of the Byzantine tradition prescribed both spiritual and bodily disciplines, including fast days and food-abstinence days aimed at cleansing both the mind and the body. The Byzantine Great Fast of Lent was sort of a Divine Spring Housecleaning for spiritual and health purposes.

The best advice to a dieter: No thyself.

–Lois Ward, Longmont, Colorado

The early Byzantine Christian liturgists were keenly aware that both Jesus and his disciples fasted occasionally, and they understood the health benefits of short fasts and food abstinences, mainly from fattening and artery-clogging animal products and sweets.

The Great Fast had the effect of promoting regularity and controlling unhealthy weight-gain. The early Greek clergy were clearly prevention-minded and concerned about the health of their congregations.

"Lent is like going to a party," explained Bishop Paul Chomnycky, O.S.B. Ukrainian Catholic Bishop of Stamford, Connecticut. "We spend 40 days getting clean and getting dressed for the party celebrated on Easter."

Here are some readings Fr. Miles found in the Byzantine Lenten liturgies:

"Oh people, let us welcome the Great Fast with joy..."

*"In Your compassion, grant that we may spend the
season of the joyful Fast in profound peace."*

*"O Savior, set me free, that with great joy
I may sing in praise of Your merciful love."*

These early Greek liturgists certainly had the gift of poetry, but they also had a keen understanding of the relationship between body and mind and the importance of ridding the body of accumulated toxins from time to time.

Modern Eastern Rite Christians are more inclined to favor the feast days over the fast days during Lent. But the Byzantine Lenten Great Fast is evidence that the early Christians were keenly aware of health matters and prevention. The annual Great Fast was a curb on one of the seven deadly sins—gluttony.

The first day of Lent in the Orthodox Church is called "Clean Monday." "This is the day that we're not supposed to have meat or dairy products," according to Fr. Demetrios Kavadas of the Assumption Greek Orthodox Church in St. Clair Shores, Michigan. Orthodox believers are called to abstain from meat and dairy products during the 40 days of Lent prior to Easter.

The 20 Greek doctors of the third century, who were referred to as the "unmercenary physicians" because they never charged their patients a fee, insisted that their patients follow the fast days of the Orthodox Church.

Foremost among these physicians, who were later canonized as saints by both the Orthodox and Catholic Churches, were St. Cosmas and St. Damian. Cosmas and Damian were Greek brothers who studied medicine in the Hippocratic schools.

They are reputed to have healed their patients with medicinal herbs, a diet of healthful foods, measured exercise, spiritual counseling, and prayer. They are said to have cured all kinds of illnesses, but they believed that their patients were cured by the grace of God.

Their enemies finally fed them to the sharks.

Another Greek physician, Panteleimon, is venerated as the patron saint of physicians. St. Panteleimon is often shown in icons holding medical instruments and medicinal herbs. A physician to Emperor Maximian, he was converted by a Christian priest, and he dedicated his skills in healing to Christ. He was denounced to the emperor as a believer in Christ, arrested, and executed by sword in A.D. 305.

After eating an entire bull, a mountain lion felt so good he started roaring. He kept it up until a hunter came along and shot him. The moral: When you're full of bull, keep your mouth shut.

–Will Rogers

Devotion to the martyred Panteleimon spread far and wide in the early church. In 532 A.D., Justinian I rebuilt a church that had been dedicated to Panteleimon at an earlier date.

Today, the Greek Orthodox monks of the centuries-old monastery of Mount Athos still follow "The Great Fast" of Lent and the health advice of the Greek "unmercenary physicians" of long ago.

A CBS *60 Minutes* documentary on the monks of Mount Athos reported that the monks have a remarkable longevity, and "there is no evidence of cancer, heart disease, or Alzheimer's among them."

The monks eat simply—fresh vegetables, fruits, and grains, which they grow themselves in organic gardens, and fish. They do physical chores and walk everywhere. They adhere to the Orthodox Church's fast days and food-abstinence days and liturgical days, and they pray constantly.

"Christian healing is not a fad of the twentieth century," *The Orthodox Weekly Bulletin* observed recently. "Great Christian healers were known in the church in ancient times, and their loving sacrifice on behalf of the sick has been an inspiration for many."

A Greek Orthodox priest complained to *The Joyful Noiseletter* not long ago that many Orthodox parishioners in America are no longer observing these ancient traditions and also are leading very sedentary lifestyles. As a result, he said, they are not as healthy as the parishioners in the old country who still observe them and are more physically active in their daily lives.

"Many of these folks, including priests, are getting to Heaven sooner than they expected," the priest said. "God made the body to be used, and he didn't command us to congest it with junk foods."

In the Age of Obesity, contemporary Christianity has weakened Lent by ignoring the health benefits of short fasts and food abstinences, and being content with "giving up candy" or "giving up meat on Fridays."

Occasional short fasts for the benefit of mind and body have been recommended by all religions. Many of the Hebrew prophets prayed and fasted. Ramadan, the ninth month of the Muslim year, a period of daily fasting from sunrise to sunset, was intended to achieve the same health benefits as the old Byzantine Lenten Great Fast.

Lenten Fasting and Feasting

Rev. James A. Gillespie, a retired Presbyterian minister in Charlerio, Pennsylvania, suggested a list of things to fast from and to feed on during Lent:

Fast from gossip;
Feast on the Gospels.

Fast from junk foods;
Feast on the Bread of Life.

Fast from bad news;
Feast on "The Good News."

Fast from darkness;
Feast on the Light.

Fast from the secular;
Feast on the sacred.

Fast from despair;
Feast on hope.

Fast from revenge;
Feast on forgiveness.

Fast from tears of sorrow;
Feast on tears of joy.

Fast from getting;
Feast on giving.

Fast from complexities;
Feast on simplicities.

Fast from horror;
Feast on humor.

Fast from listlessness;
Feast on laughter.

Benjamin Franklin's *Poor Richard's Almanack* included health maxims for the American colonists and was distributed free by clergy to poor parishioners.

"If you would live long, live well; for folly and wickedness shorten life."

"Eat to live, and not live to eat."

"To lengthen thy life, lessen thy meals."

"Many dishes, many diseases."

"Eat few suppers and you will need few medicines."

"I saw few die of hunger; of eating—100,000."

Chapter 7

John Wesley: Prophetic Health Crusader

John Wesley (1703–1791), the founder of the Methodist Church, was a great preacher who had a keen sense of humor and insisted that his followers follow Jesus' instructions to "be of good cheer."

Wesley was adept at using humor to put down hecklers and detractors. He often rode on horseback to Methodist gatherings.

One day on a narrow road, he met an arrogant judge, also on horseback, coming in the other direction. The judge refused to budge, saying, "I shall not give the road to a fool."

"But I will," replied Wesley, calmly reining his horse off the road.

More importantly, Wesley was greatly concerned with health issues facing the clergy and general public in both England and America. And he was prophetic on many health matters.

If the body is feeble, the mind will not be strong

–Thomas Jefferson

He published a book, *Primitive Physick*, with practical health tips that pastors and plain people could understand. He encouraged pastors to strive to be both spiritually and physically fit, and to instruct church members in a healthy lifestyle. The book became a best-seller in both England and America. He marveled at the good health of Americans, and attributed it to "their continual exercise, universal temperance," and a natural diet.

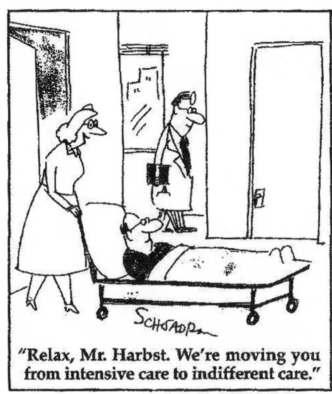

"Relax, Mr. Harbst. We're moving you from intensive care to indifferent care."

from *JoyfulNoiseletter.com*
©Harley L. Schwadron

Were Wesley still alive today, I suspect he would say that the Americans of his time were healthier than modern-day Americans. And he would be pilloried by many in today's medical establishment.

But the fact remains that the Americans of Wesley's time ate natural, organic, fresh foods—free of pesticides, preservatives, hormones, et al. They lived on slow foods, not fast foods, and breathed clean air and drank clean water.

In his book's preface, Wesley wrote: "The power of exercise, both to preserve and restore health, is greater than can well be conceived; especially in those who add temperance thereto... and steadily observe that kind and measure of food whose experience shows to be most friendly to health and strength."

Joy Burt Conti, a nurse in Mt. Lebanon, Pennsylvaniass, finds much value in Wesley's writings on health matters, as do an increasing number of physicians and medical researchers who consider Wesley prophetic.

The body is your temple. Keep it pure and clean for the soul to reside in.

–B.K.S. Lyengar, *Yoga: The Path to Holistic Health*

Conti, who chairs the Health as Wholeness Team of the Western Pennsylvania Conference of the United Methodist Church, observed in *Cross and Flame,* a Conference publication, that Wesley recommended a diet close to vegetarian (with modest amounts of animal food) and drinking a lot of water.

He saw the importance of good ventilation and sanitation, and suggested clergy should get open-air exercise three hours a day by walking or horseback riding, practice moderation in eating, and get sufficient sleep.

"The air we breathe is of great consequence to our health," Wesley wrote. "Everyone who would preserve health should be as clean as possible in their houses, clothes, and furniture."

On diet, Wesley commented:

"The great rule of eating and drinking is to suit the quality and quantity to the strength of our digestion; to take always such a sort and such a measure of food as is light and easy on the stomach."

"For studious persons, about eight ounces of animal food, and 12 of vegetable, in 24 hours, is sufficient."

"Eat very light suppers, and that two or three hours before going to bed."

"Water is the most wholesome of all drinks; quickens the appetite, and strengthens the digestion most."

Among his remedies, he praised onions and cinnamon. On exercise, Wesley commented:

"A due degree of exercise is indispensably necessary to health and long life."

"Walking is the best exercise for those who are able to bear it; riding for those who are not. The open air, when the weather is fair, contributes much to the benefit of exercise."

"We may strengthen any weak part of the body by constant exercise."

Wesley could also be entertaining. One of his remedies for a headache: "Hold a live puppy constantly on the belly."

Wesley sharply criticized those doctors who "in the pursuit of profits, produce mixtures of medicines that become useless through their opposite interactions and, which joined together, destroy life."

Wesley was also keenly aware of the spiritual side of good health. He wrote:

> "The passions have a greater influence upon health than most people are aware of. All violent and sudden passions dispose to, or actually throw people into acute diseases. The slow and lasting passions, such as grief and hopeless love, bring on chronic diseases. Till the passion which causes the disease is calmed, medicine is applied in vain.

> "Above all, add to the rest that old unfashionable medicine— prayer... the love of God is the sovereign remedy of all miseries (and) effectually prevents all the bodily disorders the passions introduce, by keeping the passions themselves within due bounds; and by the unspeakable joy and perfect calm, serenity, and tranquility it gives the mind; it becomes the most powerful of all the means of health and long life."

Wesley once suggested than the ideal physician would be a pastor knowledgeable about health, prevention, and medical matters.

Wesley lived simply and methodically and was never idle if he could help it. Like his Savior, he died poor. He was 88.

Ellen White

In the 19th century, another health reformer, Ellen White, the founder of the Seventh-Day Adventist Church, recommended a dietary and physical fitness program very similar to John Wesley's. White said she got her health and prevention ideas directly from God in her trances. Although she was raised a Methodist in her youth, you would have difficulty finding any evidence that White ever gave Wesley any credit for his health reform ideas.

There is an all-too-human reluctance among health reformers to credit the pioneers who went before them.

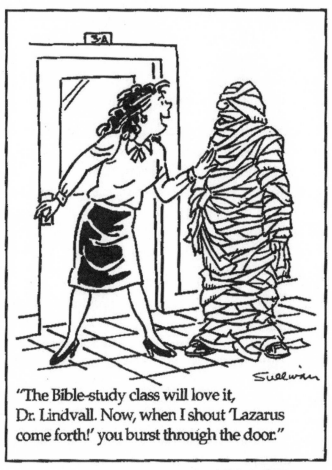

"The Bible-study class will love it, Dr. Lindvall. Now, when I shout 'Lazarus come forth!' you burst through the door."

from *JoyfulNoiseletter.com*
©Ed Sullivan

Chapter 8

Uncle Tom's Cabin Author Was Also a Health Reformer

Harriet Beecher Stowe (1811–1896)—famed for her book *Uncle Tom's Cabin*—campaigned just as passionately and humorously for good health, good nutrition, and good ventilation in churches, seminaries, and trains. She not only campaigned to free the slaves but also to free people from unhealthy habits that were causing their diseases.

In 1866, this remarkable woman contributed an article to *The Atlantic Monthly* by the intriguing title, "Bodily Religion: a Sermon on Good Health." She wrote:

> "The foul air generated by one congregation is locked up by the sexton for the use of the next assembly; and so gathers and gathers from week to week, and month to month, while devout persons are ready to tear their hair because they feel stupid and sleep in church.
>
> "Revivals of religion, with ministers and the people who take most interest in them, often end in periods of bodily ill-health and depression (because) of people breathing poison from each other's lungs.
>
> "The proper ventilation of their churches and vestries would remove that spiritual deadness of which their prayers and hymns complain.
>
> "In contrast, a man hoeing his corn out on a breezy hillside is bright and alert, his mind works clearly, and he feels interested in religion.

"The want of suitable ventilation on schoolrooms, offices, courtrooms, churches, law schools, medical schools, and theology schools is something simply appalling. Of itself it would answer the question why so many thousand glad, active children come to a middle life without joy."

Mrs. Stowe, her husband, Congregationalist Pastor Calvin Stowe, and her brother, Congregationalist preacher Henry Ward Beecher (also renowned for his wit), were among many Christians who led a health reform movement in the mid-19th-century. Like Ellen White and Methodism's John Wesley, their focus was on prevention.

At the day of Judgment, we shall not be asked what we have read but what we have done.

–Thomas á Kempis

Mrs. Stowe, the mother of five children, wrote articles for magazines to supplement her husband's meager pastor's salary. After her son, Charlie, became ill and died in 1849, she became keenly interested in helping people live healthy lifestyles.

She wrote: "Like the principles of spiritual religion, the principles of physical religion are few and easy to understand: an old medical apothegm personifies the hygienic forces as Doctor Air, Doctor Diet, Doctor Exercise, and Doctor Quiet. (*The Joyful Noiseletter* would add Doctor Laughter to that list.)

"The return to the great primitive elements of health—clean water, clean air, and simple, fresh food, with a regular system of exercise—has brought to many a jaded, weary, worn-down human being the elastic spirits and the sound sleep of a little child."

Chapter 9

The Loneliness of the Dining Room Table

By Rev. Paul Lintern

(Rev. Paul Lintern, a longtime consulting editor to *The Joyful Noiseletter*, is the pastor of two Lutheran congregations in Mansfield, Ohio. He recently bought a "chome" [church home] and lives there to help it stay vibrant as a worship center and meal site for the needy.)

I am your dining room table. I last saw you in November of 1995, the last time you hosted the family for Thanksgiving.

Listen, I know that eating together is passé (as is the word "passé"), and I know you don't need to sit to devour pizza, but I miss your company.

Back when I belonged to your great-grandmother and her siblings, I heard important family discussions around me, thanks to the three leaves that expanded me around my middle. (Those are the three wooden planks that are gathering dust in the back of the garage today.)

When your grandmother got married, I was their present from her parents. It tickled me to have your mother mix things and knead things, and the delicious, nutritious, healthy things you enjoyed growing up. I was there every day, supporting breakfast, lunch and dinner.

I miss those slow-food days, and all the table talk, the jokes, the laughter, and discussions. I could hear love in arguments and bonding in meaningless banter. I even sensed peace in the midst of six conversations going on at once.

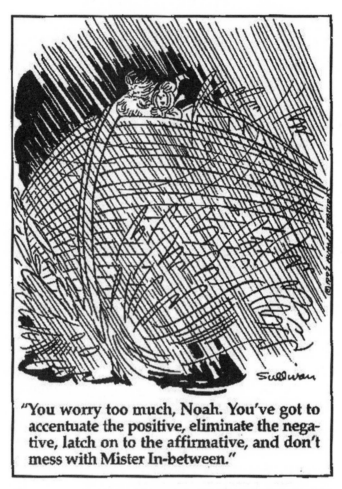

"You worry too much, Noah. You've got to accentuate the positive, eliminate the negative, latch on to the affirmative, and don't mess with Mister In-between."

from *JoyfulNoiseletter.com*
©**Ed Sullivan**

And whenever the whole family joined hands and bowed their heads and prayed together, there was something complete. I wonder how many people were comforted or encouraged or healed by that simple act.

I smiled when your mother brought "the right one" about six different times before she brought your father to dinner. Actually, he was my choice, too, because he never spilled anything on me or stuck gum under me.

I helped to make model ships with your grandpa and your Uncle Jim. I sat in on important financial decisions about the house, the job, and life in general.

It just seemed to me that where the whole family came together, magical things happened. I just sensed that when there was a complete set of ears at the table, there also was a full circle of caring.

When I was passed on to you after grandma's death, I hoped to help you recapture those special moments you must have remembered growing up, even if your parents drifted away from me.

Money will buy a fine dog, but only kindness will make him wag his tail.

–Bobbe Lyon, addiction counselor, Maitland, Florida

Since that last Thanksgiving, I have been moved to seven different homes, each one stirring in me the hope of a return to those home-cooked meals. Instead, it seems I am a collecting point, instead of a conversation point.

I will dutifully serve as a warehouse, if that is what you want. I'll collect everything you place on me—junk mail, homework, tangled piles of electronic chargers, scrapbook projects, gym shoes, and potato chip bags.

But I must admit I do miss the time when communication was face-to-face, when people voiced their concerns rather than texted them, and shared smart conversation without smart phones, when the only things we tweeted were whistles, and socials had nothing to do with media.

Just for kicks, because I love you folks, all of you, why don't you let me host you for a meal? The whole family? The whole meal? Looking at each other and bowing heads, only for prayer—not for checking cell phones.

You provide the food and drinks and table service. I will provide, well, me.

It may seem a little odd, but I suspect that you will be surprised by how pleasant the experience is—no television, no Wi-Fi, no cell phone, no i-Anything, no tweets. No telling what will happen.

Yes, it will take a while to clean me off, but even that is worth the effort every so often.

Just try it. And if you don't find it to be a family-building activity, then you can just table the idea.

"Slow Food" Days

A young friend asked me the other day, "What was your favorite fast food when you were growing up?"

"We didn't have fast food when I was growing up," I replied. "All the food was slow."

"Seriously, where did you eat?" he asked.

"It was a place called 'home,'" I explained.

"Mom cooked every day and when Dad got home from work, we sat down together at the dining room table and prayed before eating. My mother saw to it that we always had healthy, fresh foods on the table. And if I didn't like what she put on my plate, I was allowed to sit there until I did like it."

My young friend was laughing so hard I didn't tell him the part about how I had to have permission to leave the dinner table.

—Author unknown, via John Compere,
Kalamazoo, Michigan

Chapter 10

The Dietary Healing of a Baptist Doctor and a Baptist Pastor

Dr. Russell's "Bible Diet"

D r. Rex Russell had impressive credentials. He interned at the Mayo Clinic and became a radiologist on the staff at Sparks Regional Medical Center in Fort Smith, Arkansas. A member of the First Baptist Church in Fort Smith, he also raised cattle on his Arkansas farm.

So how did a Southern Baptist, cattle-raising, Mayo-Clinic-trained radiologist come to study and recommend what might be called "Dr. Russell's Bible Diet?"

As a young man, Russell had been a strapping football player on the Oklahoma State University team, whose bruises were nursed by Dr. Don Cooper, who was the team physician then.

In 1976, Russell's long-standing diabetes was worsening. He also was suffering from chronic abscesses, arthritis, swelling in his legs, and deterioration of his arteries, eyesight, and kidneys. He said:

"Because I'm a doctor, I searched for medical answers with many physicians but only experienced continued illness and confusion.

"One evening in desperation I pulled a Bible off the shelf. I happened to come across Psalm 139:14, where the Psalmist praises God because 'I am fearfully and

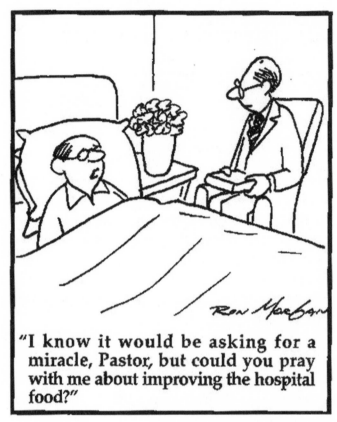

"I know it would be asking for a miracle, Pastor, but could you pray with me about improving the hospital food?"

from *JoyfulNoiseletter.com*
©Ron Morgan

wonderfully made.' I said: 'If we are so wonderfully made, why am I so sick? God, why didn't You give us a way to be healthy?'"

He received this answer: "Rex, have you really read my Instruction Book?"

Dr. Russell began to study the physiology of faith. Searching the Bible, he discovered not only spiritual laws related to health, but also dietary and physical principles which he began to apply. After four years, this dramatic change in lifestyle resulted in the recovery of his health.

Although he still was dependent on insulin, he never again had an abscess or symptoms of arthritis. He regained 20/20 vision. His overall health improved in every respect, he said.

Meanwhile, Dr. Russell studied a lot of ongoing medical research which, he said, confirmed that many of the dietary recommendations and restrictions found in the Old and New Testament have a scientific basis.

In 1998, he wrote a book—*What the Bible Says about Healthy Living* (Regal Books)—which became a bestseller. Dr. Russell was also a consulting editor to *The Joyful Noiseletter*, which featured his book in *JN's* catalog.

To improve your physical and mental health and lift your spirits, Dr. Russell recommends that you add to your diet many of the natural foods which the folks in the Old and New Testament ate, while avoiding the foods that they avoided or ate sparingly. He also recommends doing what those Biblical folks did—an occasional short fast.

In the Foreword to the book, Joe S. McIlhaney, MD, writes: "Rex Russell is one of the funniest people I know. He has used his good humor, his medical expertise, and his knowledge of scripture to help us learn what can enable us to have good health." His book explores both the scriptural and medical bases for the lifestyle changes he recommends.

Although he was not a vegetarian, this physician/cattleman believes "most people in the United States would benefit from decreased consumption of meats. Eating too much meat—both unclean meat and super-charged, chemical-enhanced, over-processed clean meat—can cause illness," he says.

Only 5% of his daily calories come from meat, he said.

Living in the middle of catfish country, Dr. Russell also recommends that people avoid catfish, as well as pork.

The folks in the Bible, he says, ate meat sparingly, and considered meat "a celebration food," eaten only for special occasions, such as the return of a prodigal.

In a chapter titled, "Mom was Right: Eat Your Fruits and Veggies," Dr. Russell recommends a diet with plenty of fresh fruits and vegetables, grains, seeds, and beans—basically, the kind of natural diet that those Mediterranean folks were eating in Biblical times and are, more or less, eating today.

Eat some garlic, too. Medical research, he says, has shown that garlic lowers bad cholesterol levels significantly, lowers high blood pressure, and protects people from infections.

Another prominent Biblical food, olive oil, has been shown by medical studies to have a beneficial effect on health, especially in preventing hardening of the arteries.

"The lifestyles of the young Hebrew Daniel and his friends provide great examples of the healthful qualities of vegetables and of eating according to God's law," Dr. Russell observes.

Carried into Babylonian captivity, Daniel and his friends were selected to serve the king in the palace. However, Daniel declined to eat the luxurious foods of the palace and received permission to eat only vegetables, lentils, and water.

"At the end of 10 days, Daniel and his friends looked healthier and better nourished than any of the young men who ate the royal food (Daniel 1:15, 20)," says Russell.

Dr. Russell recommends three principles which he believes will improve a person's health. "They are not a cure-all," he says, "but I believe they will help all."

1. Eat the foods God created for you.

2. As much as possible, eat foods as they were created, before they are changed into nutrient-deficient or toxic products.

3. Avoid food addictions. Don't let any food or drink become your god.

One part of Russell's regimen for healthy living is periodic fasting, also recommended in both the Old and New Testaments. Fasting, he believes, can help eliminate addictions and improve a person's overall physical and mental health.

"The mental benefits of fasting," he says, "include a calming effect, the ability to focus on priorities, and a generalized improvement in mental functioning. Fasting can give the body time to clear itself of toxic productions. And eating things designed for food in their purest form could be great for the mind."

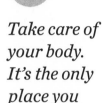

Take care of your body. It's the only place you have to live.

–Jim Rohn

He observes that "heart attacks were a medical oddity in the 1920's" and cancer was not nearly as prevalent as it is today.

Down through the centuries, periodic fasting and periodic abstinence from animal products also have been recommended by the Eastern Orthodox Church, the Catholic Church, various monastic traditions, and Protestant groups like the Seventh Day Adventists. But many of the clergy and laypeople of all denominations have not always taken these admonitions seriously, even during Lent.

The Eastern Orthodox theologian Bishop Kallistos Ware writes:

> "Until the 14th century, most Western Christians, in common with their brethren in the Orthodox East, abstained during Lent not only from meat but from animal products such as eggs, milk, butter, and cheese.

In East and West alike, the Lenten fast involved a severe physical effort. But in Western Christendom over the past 500 years, the physical requirements of fasting have been steadily reduced, until by now they are little more than symbolic. The Orthodox world in our time is also beginning to follow the same path of laxity."

Interestingly, Detroit Archbishop Adam J. Maida recently proposed that the church reinstitute abstention from meat on Fridays for American Catholics as a prayer for life issues, and 280 bishops have endorsed Maida's proposal. (We have known four overweight, under-exercised bishops who have died at comparatively young ages in the past five years.)

Dr. Russell has three other suggestions to improve one's health:

1. Exercise regularly. "The Bible says: 'By the sweat of your brow you will eat your food.' (Gen 3:19) Because most of us no longer toil in the fields for our food, physical exercise should be substituted. It is my belief that we need enough exercise to work up a sweat six days a week."

2. Don't forget to smile. "Both the giver and the receiver of a smile benefit through the release of prostaglandins. These substances help balance the hormonal functions of the body."

3. Everything in moderation (so said the Apostle Paul).

This physician, fascinated by the relationship of mind and body, raised the same question that the Apostle Paul asked 2,000 years ago, but which many modern-day clergy and laypeople have stopped asking: "Do you not know that your body is a temple of the Holy Spirit, who is in you, whom you have received from God?"

Rev. Malkmus' "Hallelujah Diet"

About the same time, Rev. Dr. George H. Malkmus, a well-known longtime Baptist pastor in New York, North Carolina, Florida, and Tennessee, authored a book titled *Why Christians Get Sick* (Destiny Image Publishers).

At the age of 42, Rev. Malkmus was told he had colon cancer. He wondered: "How could this be?" He was a Christian and a pastor who had dedicated his life to the Lord.

Not willing to accept this cancer as "God's will" for his life, like Dr. Russell, Rev. Malkmus began an intensive biblical and scientific study of health matters.

He wondered: "Could this sickness be because of 'sin' in my own life?" But he had known a Christian leader who had suffered a stroke, a Christian publisher who had a heart attack, the founder of a Christian college who suffered from senility, a Christian missionary and his own mother who had died of cancer. He had seen good Christians die in the prime of life.

Rev. Malkmus began to attend a nutritional institute in Florida, and put into practice the things he was taught on diet, exercise, and lifestyle changes.

Like Jack LaLanne, Rev. Malkmus began living on a 100% raw fruit and vegetable vegan diet. "Almost immediately unbelievable things started to happen in my body," he said. His health improved dramatically, and in time he was healed of his colon cancer. His blood pressure dropped from 150/90 to 110/70. His allergies departed, his sinuses cleared up, his eyesight improved, he stopped suffering from constipation and colds, and his energy improved dramatically.

Like Dr. Russell, Rev. Malkmus searched the Bible for answers and arrived at the same conclusions.

Malkmus noted that his grandparents were farm people, living a simple life of hard work and eating primarily simple meals prepared from the fresh food raised in their own gardens and orchard. Both remained strong and active into their 80's.

Prior to World War II, there was very little use of insecticides in the growing of food. Now, over one billion pounds of insecticides are sprayed or dusted on the food Americans consume each year. And it is very difficult to wash off or remove these poisons. It's also hard to find prepared food that doesn't contain chemical preservatives, artificial colorings and flavorings, etc. The meat being raised today is also different from the meat of his grandparents' day, he wrote. All sorts of drugs are being added to the animals' food and drink, like antibiotics to keep them well and growth hormones to cause them to grow faster.

Every man is the building of a Temple called his body.

–Henry David Thoreau

Malkmus also observed that fast food restaurants are on every corner. "Many mothers," he said, "feel that these fast foods are a convenience and a blessing because they require less time for preparation. But," he added, "are they a blessing, or are they helping contribute to the multitude of physical problems plaguing the families of today?"

Though they have knowledge of spiritual matters, "Christians," Malkmus wrote, "are often lacking in knowledge concerning the relationship between food, nutrition, lifestyle, and health."

"Baptists are often extremely fatalistic when it comes to sickness. They pray very sincerely for healing. But if prayers and the efforts of the medical profession don't bring healing, then the sickness is accepted as the 'will of God.' But in over 30 years of association with Baptists, I have not seen them, as a group, to have any better health than non-Baptists." (The same thing could be said about parishioners in other denominations.)

Malkmus added: "Christians should have open minds. Sadly, though many Christians close their minds to anything different from what their minds are programmed with, often ignorant of the truth, foolishly substituting opinions, theories, tradition, and blind belief for true knowledge."

Are many Christians of all faith traditions simply ignorant of the teachings of the Christian health reformers of the past in Catholic, Eastern Orthodox, and Protestant churches?

Too many Christians are dying in the pews today.

Not surprisingly, like Jack LaLanne, Rev. Malkmus was attacked as a "quack" by some professionals. That's the typical response when someone dares to challenge the views of the well-heeled health and theological establishment. You might even get crucified.

Dr. Russell, who had impressive credentials as a Mayo Clinic physician and radiologist, and who was saying the same things as Rev. Malkmus, was not pilloried as a quack.

Different treatments help or heal different folks. And if an unconventional treatment helps or heals someone, why should anyone complain? We should rejoice. Unconventional treatments also have a way of becoming, in time, conventional treatments.

"Once upon a time, moderation in all things was the maxim by which most people tried to live their lives. Today moderation is merely boring. Extreme is the virtue of the cool, as well as of the populace. Judging from the girths ambling among America's sidewalks, few appetites go unattended. Likewise in the political realm, passions roam unbridled. In an environment where talk radio and cable TV set the tone of discourse, dispassion and facts give way to heat and opinion. Such does not bode well for a nation in trouble."

– Columnist Kathleen Parker

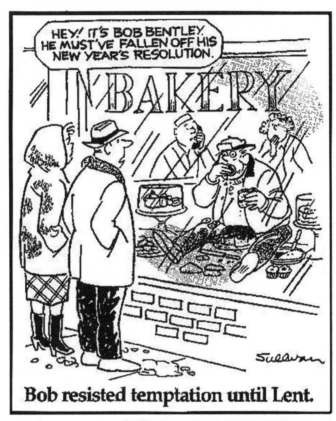

from *JoyfulNoiseletter.com*
©Ed Sullivan

Chapter 11

Overdosing on Sugar

"Sugar in the morning, sugar in the evening, sugar at supper-time." These lyrics were popularized by the McGuire Sisters in a 1948 song, "Sugartime." The McGuire Sisters were talking about sweethearts, but the 1950s were also the time that the food industry began adding sugar to many processed products, which experts in two documentary films say has resulted in an epidemic of obesity, diabetes, and associated health problems in America and worldwide.

Two extraordinary documentaries placed the blame mainly on increased consumption of sugar put into processed foods and soda pop: *Fed Up*, coproduced by Stephanie Soechtig and Katie Couric, the narrator, and *That Sugar Film* produced by Australian filmmaker Damon Gameau.

But the *Fed Up* and *That Sugar Film* documentaries were preceded in 1975 by the best-selling book, *Sugar Blues*, by William Duffy, the husband of movie legend Gloria Swanson. The book has sold over 1.6 million copies.

I met Duffy in the 1960's in New York when I was at a board meeting of the Huxley Institute for Biosocial Research. Duffy was still single then, an editor of *The New York Post*, and writing an English translation of *We Are All Sanpaku* by the Japanese author George Ohsawa, founder of the macrobiotic diet and philosophy.

Duffy, who had been ailing, said the macrobiotic diet had restored his health. The macrobiotic diet recommended by Oshawa featured brown rice as a staple food, fresh local vegetables and fruits, and the avoidance of processed foods and most animal products.

John Lennon and Gloria Swanson, who had been a vegetarian and health food advocate since her silent screen days, followed the macrobiotic diet.

What I most remember about my meeting with Duffy was his insistence that you could tell the health of a person by looking at the whites of his/her eyes. *Sanpaku* refers to a traditional Japanese diagnosis whereby eyes can be seen to present a white area on each side of the Iris. It is considered a sign of extreme fatigue, or the person may be accident prone or in poor health. (It reminded me of the old English proverb, sometimes attributed to Shakespeare: "The eyes are the windows of the soul.")

Ohsawa had also expressed concern that the introduction of refined sugar into the Japanese diet had brought with it Western diseases.

Duffy later authored his book, *Sugar Blues*, considered a dietary classic praised by John Lennon, who said he did not want his son to become a "sugar junkie." The book compared refined sugar made from sugar cane and sugar beets to drugs. It called sugar "the sweetest poison of all," and noted that it is a prime ingredient in countless food products from cereal to soup. It claimed that sugar was consumed at the rate of 100 pounds per every American annually, and it was as addictive as nicotine. The book said that sugar consumption was the cause of obesity, diabetes, a variety of physical ailments, and "the sugar blues"—"a state of depression or melancholy overlaid with anxiety."

Gloria Swanson was a long-time member of the Lutheran Church and often campaigned for school prayer as well as for health foods. After Duffy became Swanson's sixth husband in 1976, the couple traveled the world promoting *Sugar Blues*.

Swanson died at age 84; Duffy died at age 86.

> *What fools indeed we mortals are, to lavish care upon a car, with ne'er a bit of time to see, about our own machinery!*
>
> –John Kendrick Bangs

Damon Gameau's *That Sugar Film* follows in the footsteps of Morgan Spurlock's hit documentary, *Super Size Me*, in which a healthy Spurlock made himself sick by eating only fast foods from McDonald's.

Gameau didn't gorge himself on candy and ice cream. He simply ingested the equivalent of 40 teaspoons of sugar a day by eating foods that most people think are healthy—yogurt, power bars, assorted sauces, and cereals.

Sugary Mood Swings

Gameau still gained weight, experienced mood swings, and his blood work became abnormal. When he came to America, he interviewed a teenage boy whose teeth are all rotted from drinking soda pop. He also interviewed many medical and nutritional experts who claimed that sugar calories are worse than other calories, are addictive, and can affect our ability to think.

The problem, the experts said, started in the 1950s, when the McGuire Sisters were singing "Sugartime," and when the medical profession concluded that fat was the main culprit in the increase in heart disease. The food industry then started to produce "healthy" low-fat foods, but added sugar to make them taste better.

An eminent pediatrician, Dr. Robert Lustig, has appeared on PBS in a show titled, "Sweet Revenge—Turning the Tables on Processed Foods." Dr. Lusting is alarmed by what he views as an epidemic of obesity and diabetes among babies, children, and adults.

He blames "the sugar added to virtually every processed food," as well as fast foods, for the epidemic. In potato chips, he notes, you can get five different types of sugar.

The American diet has changed in the past 30 years, he says. Americans have doubled their sugar consumption in the past 60 years, mainly with soft drinks and sugar in processed foods.

Lustig maintains that "you can improve your health by cutting out fast foods and soda pop," and is critical of all the junk foods in day care centers. He recommends a low-carb diet and urges his audience to change their lifestyle.

One of his associates, Cindy Gershen, a chef who got fat and then lost a lot of weight after following Dr. Lustig's dietary advice, has written a book titled, *The Fat Chance Cookbook*, with healthy recipes without added sugar, and has a DVD called *Smart Cooking*.

In *Fed Up*, Katie Couric interviewed numerous medical doctors and nutritionists about the obesity epidemic. But its most poignant interviews were with anguished and weeping obese children (one a 15-year-old boy weighing 250 pounds, another a 13-year-old boy weighing 400 pounds.) These children were frustrated and felt helpless because they had tried to diet and exercise regularly without losing weight. They face impaired health and shorter life spans.

There has been a stunning increase in obesity among children in the past 30 years. Two decades ago, only one in ten children was overweight. Now it's one in five. One medical doctor estimated that 95% of all Americans will be obese or overweight in two decades; 30% of them will have diabetes.

"This generation will live shorter lives than their parents," one doctor said. Another doctor commented: "We're producing the world's deadliest diet and exporting it to other countries." Another doctor commented: "We have a tsunami of medical and obesity diseases."

Fed Up reports that more people will die from the effects of obesity than from starvation.

Fed Up places the blame mainly on the increased consumption of sugar put into so many processed foods, as well as soda pop. It suggests that the food industry, especially the sugar industry, have heavily financed lobbyists who have beaten back attempts by parents, schools, states, the Federal Government, and Congress to provide a healthier diet for children and to put an end to commercials for junk foods aimed at children. "Targeting children with these commercials is immoral," a doctor said.

One doctor estimated that of the 600,000 processed food items in supermarkets, 80% of them have added sugar.

Fed Up's critique of sugar consumption was subsequently supported by a study conducted by medical researchers from Tufts University, who linked the consumption of sugary drinks to an estimated 184,000 adult deaths worldwide each year.

The study found that sugary beverages would be responsible for 133,000 deaths from diabetes, 45,000 deaths from cardiovascular disease, and 6,450 deaths from cancer, *The Washington Post* reported.

> *The way he treats his body, you'd think he was renting.*
>
> –Robert Brault

Researchers collected data on deaths and disabilities from 2010 and calculated the direct effect sugar-sweetened beverages had on public health based on dietary surveys reaching more than 600,000 people. The beverages in the study included sugar-sweetened sodas, fruit drinks, sweetened iced teas, and homemade sugar drinks such as frescas.

The scientists urged people everywhere to lay off sugary drinks.

The *Fed Up* documentary views sugar as a food addiction, and big business in America. "They've placed profit ahead of public health," one doctor told Couric.

Oddly, the documentary falls short in one important respect. It pooh-poohs the traditional belief that the deadly sins—gluttony and sloth—have anything to do with the obesity epidemic.

The authorities interviewed in the documentary are willing to accept greed—another one of the deadly sins, though they do not identify it as such—as the main factor in the obesity epidemic—but not gluttony and sloth. They clearly don't feel comfortable with the language of sin.

Notwithstanding the greed of others, each of us is still in charge and can take responsibility for our own health and the health of our families by encouraging a healthy lifestyle.

This was not mentioned in *Fed Up,* but one wonders whether the old wives' tale that sweets were the tool of the devil may have given rise to the practice of giving up sweets for Lent.

All three documentaries—*Fed Up, Super Size Me,* and *That Sugar Film*—are available as DVDs and are well worth watching.

Chapter 12

The Genetically Engineered "FrankenFoods"

For over 25 years, Dr. Russell L. Blaylock, M.D., worked as a highly regarded neurosurgeon in major hospitals in the Carolinas. He taught surgical procedures to medical school students. But his medical practice took a dramatic turn after both of his parents contracted Parkinson's disease and later died when conventional medicine failed them.

Devastated, Dr. Blaylock turned his attention to medical research, searching for the causes of diseases. He discovered that the root causes of many diseases can be found in certain foods, chemicals, food additives, various toxins, and environmental hazards. He became an expert in the use of nutrition as therapy for chronic degenerative disorders.

He became the author of several best-selling natural health books and the medical editor of *The Blaylock Wellness Report*, a natural health newsletter with over 120,000 readers.

Dr. Blaylock maintains that "the root causes of many diseases, including Parkinson's, Alzheimer's, cancer, heart disease, and diabetes, may be found in GMO (Genetically Modified Organism) foods."

The problem began several decades ago, says Dr. Blaylock, when food industry biochemists discovered that they could genetically engineer plants and their seeds so that the plant would secrete higher levels of pesticides to resist insects. They did this by inserting a gene into plants like corn, soybeans, and grains. They found that it would increase farmers' crop yields.

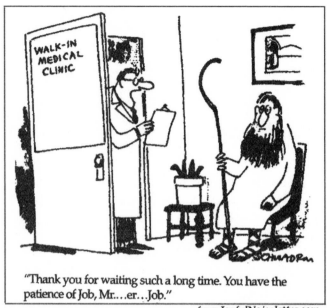

"Thank you for waiting such a long time. You have the patience of Job, Mr... er... Job."

By 2003, he said, some 60% of the crops in the U.S. were GMO crops. About 70% of the corn crops, and 90% of the soybean crops, were GMO.

Blaylock said that today 30,000 GMO foods—processed, frozen and canned—have been found in supermarkets. He believes these GMO foods are carcinogens and mainly responsible for the explosion in breast cancer and damaging kidneys and hearts.

He noted that experiments have shown that rats fed on GMO corn had double the death rates of rats that ate regular corn. They got huge cancerous tumors and died an early death.

He said that harvesters of GMO celery have reported that some workers who ate the celery experienced burning in their mouths and on their hands.

"Tens of millions of people are eating themselves sick," Dr. Blaylock said.

He said GMO food and seed manufacturers have spent millions of dollars to defeat any regulations on GMOs and opposed labeling of GMO foods.

Dr. Blaylock has authored a pamphlet titled *Dr. Blaylock's Guide to Avoiding GMO Foods* that shoppers can take with them into grocery stores to help them identify GMO foods in frozen, canned, and processed foods, and in non-organic fresh foods. The pamphlet is offered free to subscribers of *The Blaylock Wellness Report*. He also offers another pamphlet titled *What You Eat Can Kill You*.

The Blaylock Wellness Report recently promoted a video titled *Why Christians Get Sick* by Chauncey Crandall, M.D., a Christian heart specialist. Dr. Crandall raises the same questions

> *Some people have a foolish way of not minding, or pretending not to mind, what they eat. For my part, I mind my belly very studiously, and very carefully, for I look upon it, that he who does not mind his belly will hardly mind anything else.*
>
> –Samuel Johnson

that Pastor George H. Malkmus asked some years ago in his book *Why Christians Get Sick.*

"Have you ever considered why so many Christians suffer from heart disease, cancer, arthritis, digestive problems, Alzheimer's, and other health issues?" Dr. Crandall asks. "Christians appear to suffer from the same maladies as nonbelievers or members of other faiths. Does God's plan for our lives really include sickness—or is it God's will that we be healthy?"

Many Christians, Dr. Crandall says, "unwittingly violate God's natural laws for wellness. He notes that too many of his Christian patients wait until they are in really bad shape before they begin to take their health seriously—or turn to God for health." In the video, Dr. Crandall shares his strategies for living a healthy, God-centered life.

Another relentless health reformer, Brad Lemley, a longtime science writer for many publications, is the editor of a lively news-letter titled *Brad Lemley's Natural Health Solutions*, published in Baltimore, MD.

Lemley is also a robust critic of GMO foods. He also promotes the consumption of natural organic foods, especially fresh fruits and vegetables. But he parts ways with vegetarians and vegans. "Beef is good for you," he declares.

The Amish Experience

Amish farmers in southwest Michigan are moving away from using pesticides and sprays and GMO seeds, Glen Bontrager, an Amish farmer in Centreville, Michigan, told me. Bontrager raises a crop of organic corn and hay to feed his cows. He doesn't use artificial fertilizers or GMO seeds.

"The more we work at improving the quality of the soil, the better the feed and the healthier the cows and the healthier the milk," said Bontrager.

Bontrager also has fruit trees and harvests honey from his bees.

"More and more Amish farmers are going to organic farming," he said.

Another Amishman, Ivan Chupp, owner of Chupp's Herbs, a health food store in Burr Oak, Michigan, confirmed that there is a movement toward organic farming among Amish farmers.

"Medicinal herbs are also coming back big-time," Chupp said.

Alex Young, the chef and partner in Zingerman's Roadhouse in Ann Arbor, Michigan, wrote recently in the *Detroit News*:

> "People want to know more—not less—about their food. I've had countless conversations in recent years with our customers stemming from questions about how the food we serve was produced.
>
> "So it didn't surprise me when I heard about a recent survey that found 86% of Michiganians favor requiring labels for genetically engineered (GMO) foods.
>
> "Farmers and food companies have already established systems to segregate FMO and non-GMO commodities to meet the demand for non-GMO and organic products. More than 60 nations require GMO labeling, and food prices have not increased.
>
> "Survey after survey show roughly 90% of all Americans, including the vast majority of Republicans, Democrats, and Independents, want mandatory labeling laws, regardless of age, education, or race.
>
> "All Michiganians have the right to know what is in their food and how it is grown. Doesn't it make more sense to just label GMOs everywhere and trust consumers to decide for themselves?"

In his recent encyclical on the government, Pope Francis urged everyone to adopt a moral responsibility to care for our planet. "Any harm done to the environment is harm done to humanity," the Pope wrote.

That concern should extend to the impact on the health of people by miasmic environmental factors.

Too often environmental factors in illness are ignored or are pooh-poohed to appease special interests. In my hometown, Flint, Michigan, Dr. Mona Hanna-Attisha, a prominent pediatrician, reviewing blood tests at Hurley Children's Hospital, recently expressed alarm at the possible lead poisoning of the city's children who drink water pulled from the Flint River.

Residents have complained that the water from the Flint River smells, is discolored, and makes them sick, *The Detroit Free Press* reported recently.

Health officials have said that lead can lead to serious developmental problems, reducing a child's IQ, and causing serious behavioral and emotional problems.

State officials initially disputed Dr. Hanna-Attisha's test results but finally recommended that Flint reconnect to Detroit's water system.

The Free Press reported that the Flint River has been marked by decades of industrial pollution.

A Sad Case of Cross-Contamination

In 1972–73, when I was a reporter with the *Battle Creek Enquirer* in Michigan, I got a first-hand view of the destructive power of chemicals on both animal and human health when they get into the food supply.

When cows mysteriously started getting sick and dying on area dairy farms, I was assigned to cover the story. But it wasn't happening just on farms in our area; it was happening on dairy farms all over Michigan.

Cows grew thin and weak. They developed abscesses, thick hides, and elongated hooves.

The dairy farmers I interviewed were baffled, grieved, and angered over their dwindling herds and great financial losses. It took almost a year for state officials to discover the cause.

A St. Louis, Missouri company was producing both PBB (poly-brominated biophenyl), a fire retardant, and cattle feed; and bags of both were shipped to the Michigan Farm Bureau. Some of the cattle feed bags were erroneously mixed with the PBB bags, bought by farmers throughout Michigan, and fed to their dairy cows.

In those two years, about 30,000 were shot, mainly by their owners, and buried in pits to prevent further contamination. State officials quarantined 500 farms, preventing farmers from selling their cows or milk, and the Michigan dairy industry suffered huge losses.

Keeping your body healthy is an expression of gratitude to the whole cosmos—the trees, the clouds, everything.

–Thich Nhat Hanh

Forty years later, Robin Erb, *Detroit Free Press* medical editor, revisited some of the farm families and found many of them suffering from a variety of ailments. They said they were healthy prior to the PBB contamination. One woman reported that three of her grown children were plagued with health problems, and one died of leukemia at age 50.

Another farmer complained that he developed heart disease and arthritis. Still another farmer reported that many of her classmates have died or were seriously ill with a variety of diseases.

"Suddenly everything is dying and going still," she said. "There are no more mice or cats and birds anymore."

One Battle Creek area man, Jeff Jackson, Produced a short film titled *Cattlegate* about the PBB contamination.

We should be concerned about the pollution of both our water and our food supply.

Considering all the health problems created by GMO foods and the sugaring of America, one wonders how President Teddy Roosevelt, the guardian of American public health, would have responded were he alive today. No doubt he would have cracked down on the FDA he created and on the food industry and its lobbyists.

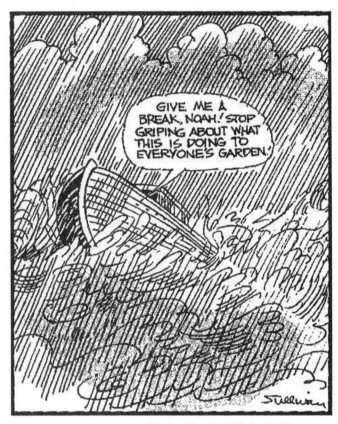

from *JoyfulNoiseletter.com*
©Ed Sullivan

Chapter 13

Medicinal Herbs for Your Mind and Body

In the past few years, *National Geographic* has published a couple of extraordinary books that focus on health. *The Joyful Noiseletter* featured in our catalog *The Blue Zones: Lessons for Living Longer from the People Who've Lived the Longest* by Dan Buettner. Another fascinating *National Geographic* book is *Nature's Best Remedies: The World of Health and Healing All Around You.*

Readers of the second book are urged to "explore the healing properties of plants, discover remedies to ailments, and uncover ways to stay healthy naturally." The book observes that "both ancient and modern health practices include the use of medicinal plants and herbs to treat a variety of ailments."

> *The body is a sacred garment.*
>
> –Martha Graham

The book also notes that certain herbs can help plummeting moods, and "medicinal herbs are a time-tested, and in some cases scientifically supported, method to support a healthy mind."

The book recommends growing your own medicinal plants in your garden, and recommends do-it-yourself container herbal gardens.

I was fascinated by the medicinal and healing properties of the herbs and vegetables described in the book because my own old-country mother grew many of them in her own organic garden and cooked wonderful meals for us with them. Being raised on these medicinal herbs as a child and as a young man, I was always healthy and bursting with energy—and rarely sick.

For centuries, families in the Mediterranean countries maintained their own organic and herbal gardens, and many still do. Mary, the mother of Jesus, also no doubt maintained her own organic and herbal garden, was probably an expert in the use of medicinal herbs, and raised Jesus on those foods.

Many of the medicinal herbs mentioned in the *National Geographic* book are common to Mediterranean diets.

Thyme, a cooking and healing herb, doubles as a spice and as a medicine. Cinnamon, as a spice, improves circulation. Garlic—"the clove that cures"—prevents and treats heart disease, reduces high blood pressure, and helps digestive complaints.

Ginger helps digestive problems. Cardamom as a spice is used to treat digestive ailments, heartburn, and constipation.

Peppermint soothes upset stomachs, improves digestion, and treats colds.

Rosemary has antibacterial, antifungal, and antiparisitic properties.

'Tis in ourselves that we are thus or thus. Our bodies are our gardens to which our wills are gardeners.

–Shakespeare, *Othello*

Parsley helps treat kidney stones and clear urinary tract disorders.

My mother also fed us fresh spinach, which nourishes the bones and wards off Alzheimer's; lots of tomatoes—full of vitamin C which is important for prostate health and lowers the risk of prostate cancer; avocadoes, a rich source of protein and vitamins; and broccoli, high in vitamins C and A.

We often had freshly made yogurt on the table. Yogurt, the book notes, is high in calcium, benefits digestion, relieves constipation, and preserves bone health.

And we usually had fresh grapes on the table. Grapes contain powerful antioxidants, lower high cholesterol and high blood pressure, and are used to treat a host of circulatory ailments.

My mother never read a book on nutrition. The nutritional wisdom she possessed had been passed down to her by word-of-mouth through the centuries by Christian mothers, who in turn had received it from the Jewish mothers who came before them.

Thanks, Mama. We miss you.

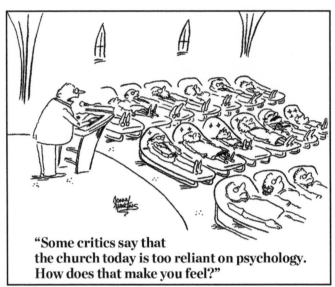

from *JoyfulNoiseletter.com*
© Jonny Hawkins

Chapter 14

The Physiology of Madness

In the 1960s, between newspaper jobs as a reporter, occasionally reporting on medical research, I met two extraordinary psychiatrists who were also biochemists and mental health reformers. One of them, Dr. Abram Hoffer, was a Canadian who was the director of psychiatric research at Fort Saskatchewan; the other. Dr. Humphry Osmond was an Englishman who had become the director of psychiatric research for the New Jersey Psychiatric Institute in Princeton.

Osmond and Hoffer for years had done extensive research together on the biochemistry of schizophrenia, alcoholism, and other psychiatric disturbances. Both of them were strong, charismatic personalities. Hoffer, a devout Jew who had been raised on a farm in Canada, had the energy and intensity of an Old Testament prophet. Osmond, a Christian, was the merry-hearted wit who could have made a living as a stand-up comic. Both were brilliant; both were physically fit.

They became good friends, whose company I greatly enjoyed. They were my "Odd Couple." When I met them, they were driving the American Psychiatric Association and the mental health establishment crazy with their sharp critiques of psychoanalysis and the myriad of costly psychotherapeutic theories and treatments of the day, which they saw as ineffective.

Osmond faithfully chronicled the ailments, real and fancied, of Winston Churchill, Samuel Johnson, and other political and literary geniuses. He had been a surgeon in the Royal Navy during World War II, and had known a couple of Churchill's personal physicians.

"His doctors always treated Churchill delicately and with a sense of humor," Dr. Osmond recalled, "because just one slip with a patient as mercurial as Winston Churchill could spell disaster."

"Churchill," Osmond said, "suffered from depressions and various ailments much of his life, but he always had the good sense to choose competent physicians who were usually witty, light-hearted, and optimistic in their style."

Osmond recalled that one of Churchill's favorite physicians, Dr. Geoffrey Marshall, was "a brilliant, witty man who cheered Churchill greatly with his amusing remarks while nursing Churchill through a bout of pneumonia in Marrakesh."

Dr. Osmond told me he is convinced that "Jesus had an excellent sense of humor and a pungent wit. If he hadn't, he could not have made such a favorable impression on publicans and sinners, and such an unfavorable impression on the religious establishment. The Gospel brought glad tidings."

Osmond and Hoffer discovered in their research that megavitamin therapy—massive doses of niacin (vitamin B3) and vitamin C—were curative or helpful in the treatment of schizophrenics and alcoholics. And in their writings and books, they relentlessly advocated this therapy as a safe and inexpensive treatment. They coauthored an extensive list of papers and books, including *The Chemical Basis of Clinical Psychiatry*.

The psychoanalysts and peddlers of antidepressants and tranquilizers were alarmed and rose up in anger with sharp criticisms of Osmond and Hoffer and their research.

In defense of their revolutionary approach to mental illness, Osmond and Hoffer assembled a board of many of the world's most respected psychiatric researchers and biochemists in a psychiatric research foundation which was to become the Huxley Institute for Biosocial Research. It was named in honor of their friends Sr. Julian Huxley, the eminent British biologist/geneticist, and his brother, the novelist Aldous Huxley.

They invited me to serve as the lay executive director of the foundation, and to be the editor of its newsletter, which I did for its first six years.

The Huxley Institute's mission was to continue to fund new research on the physiology and treatment of the serious mental illnesses. It aimed to support research in the direction no psychiatrist had gone before, unnerving many in the mental health establishment.

One Huxley Institute board member, Dr. Alan Cott, a New York psychiatrist, did a report on how Russian psychiatrists had helped many institutionalized Russian mental patients by putting them occasionally on short fasts. Ironically, short fasts were a long-standing liturgical practice of the Russian Orthodox Church.

What we feel and think are to a great extent determined by the state of our ductless glands and viscera.

–Aldous Huxley

The distinguished American biochemist Linus Pauling, who had been awarded the Nobel Prize in chemistry in 1954 and the Nobel Prize for his peace activism in 1962, also joined the scientific board of the Huxley Institute. Pauling, whom *New Scientist* called "one of the greatest scientists of all time," is the only person ever to be awarded two unshared Nobel Prizes.

Pauling promoted megavitamin therapy, and in a book he authored titled *How to Live Longer and Feel Better*, he recommended megadoses of vitamin C to treat depression, cancer, and colds. Paulings' book might have been more accurately titled *Five Fresh Oranges a Day Keeps the Psychiatrist Away*. Pauling lived to age 93.

Osmond's and Hoffer's research pointed in the direction of nutritional deficiencies in severe mental illnesses, and both psychiatrists became keenly interested in diet.

Osmond and Hoffer were pilloried by psychiatrists who depended on psychotherapy for their income; but decades later, researchers found that niacin was helpful in the treatment of Alzheimer's.

At the age of 87, Dr. Hoffer, a nutritionist as well as a psychiatrist, wrote a book titled *Hoffer's Laws of Natural Nutrition* (Quarry Press, Ontario), in which he guided readers to a more natural, primitive diet.

He sharply criticized "The Junk Food Era" of refined and processed foods. He pointed out the dietary diseases caused by low-fiber foods, high sugar and high fat consumption, vitamin and mineral deficiencies, and excessive additives.

Jesus, he observed, "lived at a time when the diet was primitive. There were no processed foods."

He wrote: "I am not Messianic on diets. Different diets may help different people. But there are benefits to a more primitive diet for everyone." (Echoes of John Wesley, but Dr. Hoffer believed in "biochemical individuality." One man's meat could very well be another man's poison, as an old saw asserted.)

Dr. Hoffer had also done a lot of research on allergies. He found that many people of Mediterranean, Asian, and African ancestry have allergies to milk and dairy products; and the allergy may be genetically based. Because for centuries their ancestors did not drink milk, they never developed the metabolic equipment to digest milk.

According to a recent study by scientists from the University of Las Palmas de Gran Canaria and the University of Granada, eating commercial baked goods and fast foods have been linked to depression. The study, published in the *Public Health Nutrition Journal*, indicated that consumers of fast foods, compared to those who eat little or none, are more likely to develop depression.

In his book, Dr. Hoffer was critical of many psychiatrists and psychologists for their ignorance of nutrition and environmental factors (such as molds and fungi in homes, which can precipitate psychiatric symptoms).

Another well-known national figure, Bill Wilson ("Bill W."), the founder of Alcoholics Anonymous, had befriended Osmond and Hoffer, was a frequent visitor to the foundation's board meetings, and an enthusiastic supporter of megavitamin therapy for alcoholics. You could buy megavitamins over the counter.

Osmond and Hoffer, in turn, were great supporters of the spiritual approach to alcoholism embodied in Alcoholics Anonymous.

Osmond and Hoffer also were admirers of the work of Dr. Thomas Kirkbride (1809–1883), the Quaker physician, health reformer, and advocate for the mentally ill. Dr. Osmond wrote a paper on how Kirkbride pioneered a plan to improve medical care for the mentally ill, designing asylum buildings which he believed were humane and promoted recovery and healing. The privacy of patients was respected, and each patient had his or her own room in buildings in lovely, rural settings.

Kirkbride believed that the mentally ill could be treated with spiritual and medical care, and many of them could be cured. He himself married a former patient.

Osmond and Hoffer were critical of the indifference and/or hostility to religion as a healing force among many in the mental health establishment—which persists today.

Osmond and Hoffer wrote an article reporting that the Quakers of the 19th century established asylums for the mentally ill in Pennsylvania that artfully combined a caring spiritual approach with a healthy diet and the best medical care of their times.

They wrote boldly that there is no evidence that America's well-endowed, well-staffed, and very costly mental health clinics and sanitariums are doing any better in healing and rehabilitating

Most psychologists treat the mind as disembodied, a phenomenon with little or no connection to the physical body. Conversely, physicians treat the body with no regard to the mind or the emotions. But the body and mind are not separate, and we cannot treat one without the other.

–Candace Pert

the mentally ill than the spiritually-oriented, inexpensive, private asylums operated by the Quakers in Pennsylvania in the 19th century. Of course, that did not endear them to the mental health establishment.

Osmond's and Hoffer's criticisms of the mental health establishment still resonate today. Its failures fill the headlines in our newspapers and on our television screens.

The Catholic bishops paid psychiatrists and therapists huge salaries to treat a small minority of pedophile priests who were seducing altar boys. The mental health professionals would report to the bishop that the pedophile was "cured," and he would be returned to his parish or assigned to another parish in another city. But he wasn't cured. And the scandal cost the Catholic Church millions in lawyer's fees, litigation, and damages.

Both the secular and the religious press typically treat the mental health establishment with kid gloves. They blamed everything on the bishops and never investigated the role of the mental health professionals in the treatment of the pedophile priests.

The news media also failed to investigate the role of the mental health professional who was treating James Holmes when the disturbed young man shot dozens of people who were watching a Batman movie in a movie house. What kind of drugs had been prescribed for Holmes? What kind of psychotherapy? Was he under psychoanalysis?

In another recent incident, Vincent Montano, 29, entered a movie theater showing "Mad Max: Fury Road" near Nashville and terrorized moviegoers with pepper spray, a pellet gun, and an ax. He was shot and killed by police.

We live in an overly medicated culture: 'A pill for every ill, and a potion for every emotion.' Certain pharmaceutical firms bear serious responsibility for promoting their products without proper safeguards.

–Fr. John Rausch,
Catholic Exponent,
Youngstown, Ohio

Montano had been committed to hospitals for psychiatric treatment at least four times, twice in 2004 and twice in 2007, police said. Again the news media failed to ask the psychiatrists who treated him any hard questions about the therapy Montano was given.

The news media also failed to investigate the role of mental health professionals who may have screened or treated the 20-year-old man before he shot and killed 26 children and teachers at Christmastime in Newtown, Connecticut.

The young man spent most of his waking hours at a computer and a flat-screen TV set in the windowless basement of his divorced parents' $600,000 home, playing violent video games across dozens of online gaming sites. In the basement, his mother had collected an arsenal of assault rifles.

The family never went to church or any house of worship. He grew up without faith or a moral compass. He lived on imported fast foods and never exercised or played with others.

The news media tends to treat the mental health establishment with kid gloves, and again failed to ask any hard questions about the kind of mental health care this disturbed young man may have been receiving. What specific antidepressants or tranquilizers were these patients on?

The mental health establishment has the perfect defense. They can, and will, call their critics crazy or quacks, or hide behind the stone wall of "doctor/patient confidentiality."

The Suicidal Hollywood Comic Culture

The news media also failed to ask any hard questions regarding the mental health establishment's treatment of the Hollywood comedians who recently killed themselves.

The tragic suicide of the enormously talented comedian Robin Williams at the age of 63 greatly distressed his friends and fans.

Williams' widow said Williams, who hanged himself in his mansion, had been struggling with depression, anxiety, and the early stages of Parkinson's disease. Previously, the comedian had suffered for years from bouts of substance abuse and alcoholism.

One report indicated that marital problems, two divorces, and money woes also took a heavy toll on Williams.

Williams' widow later claimed that it was a form of dementia, reported by the coroner, that caused her husband to hang himself.

Columnist Andrew Heller expressed puzzlement at the ongoing parade of celebrity deaths, including comedians, at comparatively young ages: "Celebrities have all the things we think we want—fame, glory, adulation, money, possessions. And it startles us when that's clearly not enough."

These celebrities also had plenty of money to be treated by expensive, top-of-the-line psychiatrists, doctors, and surgeons who could give them face-lifts as they aged.

Another prominent comedian, John Belushi, one of the funniest stars on Saturday night Live, died in 1980 at the age of 33 from an overdose of a mixture of heroin and cocaine at a party attended by Robin Williams.

Williams was devastated by his friend Belushi's death. Not long afterwards, he remarked, "Cocaine is God's way of telling you, you are making too much money."

The brilliant African-American stand-up comic, Richard Pryor, poured rum on his body and set himself on fire after free-basing cocaine and drinking 151-proof rum. He said he tried to commit suicide, but he survived burns covering more than half of his body.

Pryor, who co-wrote the movie "Blazing Saddles," was noted for his constant profanity in his acts. He was married nine times to seven different women. He died of a heart attack in 2005 at the age of 65.

Another prominent comedian, Canadian John Candy, died of a heart attack at the age of 43 after a late-night dinner. Candy was a food-addict who weighed 330 pounds and a chronic cigarette smoker. Like Belushi, he was over-weight and lived life in the fast lane.

The acid-tongued comedienne Joan Rivers died recently after a stroke and a dubious surgery. Her husband, a TV sit-com producer, had earlier committed suicide after one of his productions had been rejected.

The most recent tragedy was the death of the comedian and comedy writer Harris Wittels of a possible drug overdose at the age of 30. Wittels, best known for his work on NBC's "Parks and Recreation," died at his Los Angeles home. He had earlier talked about his struggles with drug abuse.

> *Counseling psychology essentially looks backward and inward; the child of God looks upward and forward.*
>
> –Martin and Deidre Bobgan, Santa Barbara, CA

There is also such a thing as "slow suicide." Didn't the well-heeled doctors and psychiatrists of these poor rich celebrities encourage them to live healthy lifestyles, with good nutrition, regular exercise, and sufficient sleep? Didn't they warn them that you can't continuously abuse your body with drugs, alcohol, cigarettes, junk foods, processed foods, and fast foods without serious consequences to your health?

Or did they simply treat them with other drugs—antidepressants and tranquilizers—and psychoanalysis? Did these doctors encourage their patients' belief that they could find health and happiness in drugs? These physicians should be held accountable, but the news media are too timid to ask them hard questions.

Were there no clergy around to tell them what they needed was a faith-lift, not face-lifts, and a lifestyle change?

The suicide rate in the U.S. is at a 25-year high, especially among young people. Do people really expect our children to find health and salvation in Hollywood's culture of drugs, alcohol, psychobabble, rampant egotism, and self-indulgence?

Our issues were with the doctors and therapists who treated these unfortunate comedians. Their counsel and treatments were not very helpful. Too many of us have forgotten the wisdom of the doctors, pastors, and healers of past centuries.

For centuries, until the 20th century, people with emotional and mental problems went to their pastors for spiritual counseling and to their family doctors for advice on their diet, medication, and physical health.

Starting in the early 20th century, psychiatrists began to proliferate and usurped the roles of the clergy and the family physician. Psychiatry—with its arsenal of psychoanalysis, antidepressants, and tranquilizers—became big business, but was unable to stem the epidemic of madness that spread across the land.

After reviewing the results of myriad secular psychotherapeutic techniques, two professors of psychology have concluded that nonprofessionals are just as effective, or more effective, at helping mental patients as are professionals like psychiatrists, psychologists, and social workers.

Writing in *Psychological Science*, Andrew Christensen, professor of psychology at the University of California, Los Angeles, and Ned Jacobsen, professor of psychology at Washington University in St. Louis, noted that no one in the mental health establishment is eager to fund a study comparing professional therapy with nonprofessional therapy.

Both Dr. Osmond and Dr. Hoffer out-lived many of their critics, Osmond dying at the age of 87, Hoffer at the age of 92. I feel blessed that I could count them among my friends.

Chapter 15

How to Avoid Alzheimer's

Hall of Fame broadcaster Joe Garagiola, a consulting editor to *The Joyful Noiseletter*, wrote one of the funniest books ever written about Major League baseball—*Just Play Ball*.

One of Garagiola's favorite ballplayers was his friend, the African-American pitcher Satchel Paige, whom Garagiola described as a "great philosopher."

Satchel was still pitching in the Major Leagues at age 48, and reporters once asked him how he had lasted so long. "Keep runnin' and don't look back, 'cause somebody might be gainin' on you," Satchel replied.

Garagiola noted the Apostle Paul pretty much said the same thing when he told the Philippians, "Forgetting what is behind and straining toward what is ahead, I press on toward the goal to win the prize..." Observed Garagiola: "Satchel may have been only paraphrasing Paul."

Reporters were always curious about exactly how old Satchel was. Satchel told them: "I don't know. My mama always kept the birthdays of all my brothers and sisters in the family Bible, but our goat ate the Bible."

He added: "How old would you be if you didn't know how old you are? I know 20-year-old guys with 90-year-old minds, and 90-year-old guys with 20-year-old minds."

Satchel lived to a ripe old age with his mind intact.

According to the *World Alzheimer Report*, worldwide the number of people with dementia, including Alzheimer's, will nearly triple from 47 million today to 132 million in 2050. The mental health establishment people are probably licking their chops in anticipation of this deluge of new patients.

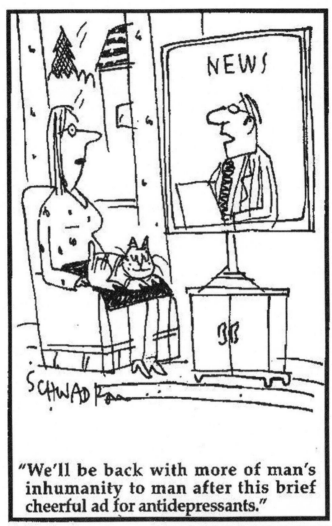

"We'll be back with more of man's inhumanity to man after this brief cheerful ad for antidepressants."

A recent medical study reported that a staggering one in three American seniors dies with Alzheimer's disease or other type of dementia. Nearly two-thirds of Americans with Alzheimer's are women.

Author Jean Carper, a nutrition specialist and former medical correspondent for CNN, gathered a variety of medical studies and published her findings in an intriguing book titled *100 Simple Things You Can Do to Prevent Alzheimer's and Age-Related Memory Loss* (Little, Brown).

"Researchers now know that Alzheimer's, like heart disease and cancer, develops over decades and can be influenced by lifestyle factors, including cholesterol, blood pressure, obesity, depression, education, nutrition, sleep, and mental, physical, and social activity," Carper reports.

Laughter is the sun that drives winter from the human face.

–Victor Hugo

"The idea that Alzheimer's is entirely genetic and preventable is perhaps the greatest misconception about the disease," says Gary Small, M.D., director of the UCLA Center on Aging.

Dr. Small recommends, among other things, "aerobic exercise (such as a brisk, 30-minute walk every day), strenuous mental activity, eating salmon and other fish, and avoiding obesity, chronic stress, sleep deprivation, heavy drinking, and Vitamin B deficiency."

This is a worthwhile book, full of many excellent health tips; but Carper interviews only modern-day medical researchers and completely ignores all of the Christian religious figures and medical doctors from centuries past who gave the same or very similar advice, without charging for it.

For instance, Carper and her experts suggest that people "follow the Mediterranean diet," and declare that diet is "a rich menu of many complex brain benefactors."

Writes Carper: "The Mediterranean diet, no matter where you live, can help save your brain from memory deterioration and dementia. Studies consistently find that what the Greeks and Italians traditionally eat is truly brain food. Following this diet—rich in green leafy vegetables, olive oil, fish, fruits, nuts, legumes, and a little vino, can cut your chances of Alzheimer's in half. Adhering most faithfully to the Mediterranean diet cuts the odds of slipping into Alzheimer's by 48%!

"Eat antioxidant-rich foods—berries, grapes, all kinds of fresh fruits and vegetables."

This is precisely the diet that the Greek "unmercenary physicians" recommended in the fourth century A.D., and what John Wesley and the early Methodists recommended in the 18th century, and what Harriet Beecher Stowe, Ellen White, the Seventh-Day Adventists, and Dr. John Harvey Kellogg recommended in the 19th century.

Science News recently reported new research on elderly Manhattan residents indicating that "people who eat a Mediterranean-style diet (rich in fresh vegetables, whole grains, and fruits) are less likely than their peers to develop Alzheimer's. And a five-year medical research study, reported recently in the *New England Journal of Medicine*, confirmed that the plant-based Mediterranean diet significantly reduced (by 30%) rates of heart attacks and strokes.

Carper's book also warns about "the dangers of meat. Too much meat primes your brain for Alzheimer's. The more meat you eat the more likely you are to have dementia."

Carper suggests that you "limit the amount of red meat you eat: beef, pork, and lamb, and particularly processed cured meats: ham, cold-cuts, hot dogs, and bacon."

So what's new? The Greek "unmercenary physicians," John Wesley, Harriet Beecher Stowe, Ellen White, Sylvester Graham,

A new study shows that women who are just a little bit overweight live longer than the men who point it out to them.

–Author Unknown

Dr. John Harvey Kellogg, Bernarr MacFadden, and Jack LaLanne said the same thing long ago.

Carper suggests cutting down on sugar. "Too much sugar creates Alzheimer's plaques in the brain," she writes.

She also warns about smoking. "Smoking can steal years of good memory," she writes. John Wesley, Ellen White, and other earlier health reformers also warned about smoking's damage to health.

St. Paul said that a *little* wine is good for the stomach. Carper says a *little* alcohol is good for the brain, but a lot of alcohol doubles the odds of developing Alzheimer's.

Carper also warns: "Know the dangers of fast foods. They wreck the body and the brain. Mountains of studies show that fatty, sugary fast foods promote heart disease, cancer, diabetes, and other diseases. It would be a miracle if they spared the brain."

"Avoid inactivity," she advises. "Enjoy exercise. It's like Miracle-Gro for aging brain cells. The more you move, the better you think. This is precisely the advice of St. Francis of Assisi, John Wesley, Harriet Beecher Stowe, Ellen White, Dr. John Harvey Kellogg, Bernarr MacFadden, and Jack LaLanne.

Carper also advises people to "practice meditation." Dr. Andrew Newberg of the University of Pennsylvania School Of Medicine recommends yoga meditation, which dramatically increases brain blood flow in older people.

Yoga is a system of physical and mental exercises developed by Hindu and Buddhist gurus, including breath control and the chanting of mantras. Many gurus also recommend a vegetarian diet.

"For the first time, we are seeing scientific evidence that meditation enables the brain to actually strengthen belief... and may even prevent neurodegenerative diseases such as Alzheimer's," Dr. Newberg said.

Carper suggests the reader "look for meditation centers in your area" (but not churches or other houses of worship) and promotes Transcendental Meditation.

The weakness of this otherwise excellent book is that it fails to mention the health and healing traditions of the Christian faith and prayer. Many Christian medical doctors, hospital chaplains, and pastors have witnessed the power of faith and prayer for many years. But this book gives short shrift to the experiences of Christian health professionals and pastors.

The author mentions that while writing her book, she took up tennis because she thought it was an excellent aerobic exercise. I have been a lifelong tennis player, but I have known good tennis players who, tragically, developed Alzheimer's at the ages of 50 and 75. Exercise helps, but there are other important factors besides exercise.

A better book is *The Blue Zones: Lessons for Living Longer from the People Who've Lived the Longest* by Dan Buettner (National Geographic).

Healthy Centenarians

With the support of *National Geographic,* Buettner led an expedition of medical scientists and health professionals from various disciplines to five areas of the world with some of the world's longest-lived people: communities on Sardinia, Okinawa, Costa Rica, Greece, and Loma Linda, CA.

They interviewed many centenarians and discovered that, despite differences in their cultures, they shared certain things in common: they had a cheerful attitude towards life and a sense of humor and laughed a lot; were serious about their faith; had strong, extended-family ties; ate a mainly plant-based diet with a focus on fresh vegetables, fruits, whole grains, beans, nuts, and fish; and stayed physically active. They did not eat fast foods, junk foods, or processed foods full of additives. They did not smoke cigarettes.

A high rate of the seniors in these five communities managed to avoid many of the diseases—like cancer, heart disease, diabetes, depression, Alzheimer's, and dementia—that are crippling and killing many Americans.

Carper's book also touched very lightly on environmental factors, which greatly concerned Dr. Hoffer and Dr. Osmond at the Huxley Institute.

A Christian medical doctor and nutritionist, Dr. Don Colbert of Lake Mary, FL, wrote recently: "Americans are exposed to more than 80,000 toxic chemicals every day, indicated by figures issued by the Environmental Protection Agency."

Doctors and scientists just don't know what the impact of all these chemicals will be on the human brain and body over the years.

Dr. Colbert and other doctors are exploring ways to eliminate toxic chemicals from your body, including an old Christian practice—occasional short fasts.

Books about doctors' and scientists' research tend to be humorless. And Carper's book entirely neglects the healing power of humor, which this book will touch on in chapter 21.

Some researchers have found that Alzheimer's patients respond favorably to humor, and some caregivers have reported that a regular prayer life is beneficial to Alzheimer's patients.

Epitaph on a pastor's monument:

Go tell the church that I'm dead,
But they need shed no tears;
For though I'm dead, I'm no more dead
Than they have been for years.

– Rev. Tal D. Bonham

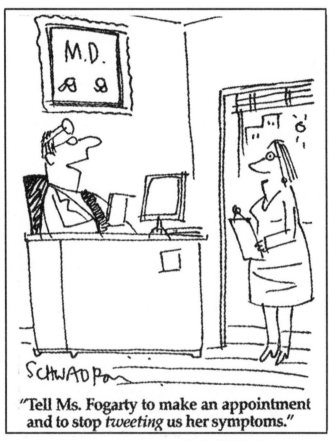

"Tell Ms. Fogarty to make an appointment and to stop *tweeting* us her symptoms."

from *JoyfulNoiseletter.com*
©Harley L. Schwadron

Chapter 16

The Church Heath Center— "Health Care Is a Mess"

"Health care is a mess, and churches can help make changes by reclaiming the biblical mandate to bring healing." That's the message of Scott Morris, M.D., a family practice physician and ordained Methodist minister who founded the Church Health Center.

Dr. Morris founded the Church Health Center in Memphis, TN, in 1987 to provide quality, affordable health care for working people and their families who are without health insurance. The Center's focus is on prevention and health education, and the interfaith concept is spreading to other cities.

Dr. Morris describes his ministry in a fascinating book titled *God, Health, and Happiness* (Barbour Publishing). This book should be in every pastor's, doctor's, nurse's, and counselor's library. It points churches in the direction they should go if they mean to be relevant in today's ailing world.

The Center has mobilized broad-based financial and volunteer support in the Memphis interfaith community, and cares for over 55,000 patients without relying on government funding. Its annual budget is about $13 million. Modest fees are charged on a sliding scale based on income and family size.

The Center has a staff of 220 people, and hundreds more volunteer their time and services. There is religious diversity with Protestants, Catholics, Jews, Muslims, Buddhists, and a Hindu Sikh, among the volunteers.

Bishop Terry Steib of the Catholic Diocese of Memphis "is a huge fan of the Center," said Marvin Stockwell, the Center's Public Relations Manager, himself a Catholic.

Janet DiLeo, a Catholic nurse who worked as a volunteer at the Center after Katrina hit New Orleans, returned to Louisiana to help start the New Orleans Faith Health Alliance, modeled after the Memphis Center. Twenty-five other cities around the country are starting similar clinics modeled after the Memphis Center.

"Efforts at health care reform fail because they avoid the essential questions of wellness," writes Dr. Morris. "The starting point is off-kilter. Our health care system is built on the premise of waiting for people to break in some way and then come through our doors, where we will use our technological wizardry to fix them.

"That's not health care. Caring for health means attending to the things that keep you well long before you break and need the door to technology. And doctors are only one part of true health care."

Dr. Morris says he values the technological advances in medicine. He himself has benefitted from a prosthetic hip that has relieved years of pain. But, he contends:

> "We have an unholy love affair with technology... Technology and business have hijacked health care: the cost of insurance, the cost of seeing doctors, the cost of medications, the cost of a hospital stay, the cost of an operation. Conversations about health care seem to be more about cost than health.
>
> "We believe that no matter what the situation, technology can solve the problem. Too many of us have the attitude that it doesn't matter how I've lived my life, what I eat, how many cigarettes I smoke, how long I sit on the couch. Technology can fix what happens even when I persist in unhealthy habits. The cost of this new technology is astronomical."

"So what system would make people healthier? Understanding what it means to be well—body and spirit. And developing behaviors and lifestyles that focus on what works, not on what is broken. That's the essence of prevention.

"The heart of a health care system focuses on keeping you well—preventing bodily breakdowns—and requires a return to the belief that caring for people's health is a helping profession, not big business."

Model for Healthy Living

The Church Health Center has developed a "Model for Healthy Living" as a tool to help people choose ways to care for their own health. This model urges individuals to take charge of their own health care and focuses on good nutrition, friends and family, emotional life, work, regular exercise, faith, cultivating a sense of humor, and medical care.

"We don't start with the doctor; we start with the 'health coach,'" says Morris.

At the Center, people come together and encourage one another in exercise, nutrition, support groups, and prayer. Dr. Morris also values humor as a healing tool.

And health improves!

The Center's attitude toward nutrition is "all things in moderation." Morris is also critical of over-indulgence in fast-foods and their contribution to the nation's epidemic of obesity that is landing a lot of people in hospitals.

The center encourages patients to exercise regularly, within their physical limitations. "Sedentary is not how God made you. You are created to move," says Morris.

People, even more than things, have to be restored, renewed, revived, reclaimed and redeemed. Never throw out anyone.

–Audrey Hepburn

Morris observes: "Our culture is full of messages that run counter to a true understanding of wellness. Don't believe everything you read—on the Internet, in TV commercials, and even in churches. Unfortunately, the church carries false messages of its own that pull us away from health, rather than toward it."

Church people who have regular feeding frenzies on fast foods and at church potlucks, who are overfed and under-exercised, are jeopardizing their health.

Morris writes:

> "One of the common fallacies still promoted in many churches is the division of body and spirit, and that you can do anything to your body because God has already given you salvation for your soul.
>
> "What happens in your body is not separate from what happens in your spirit. You honor God when you care for your body. The health care system is a mess, but you don't have to be.
>
> "Our lives are healthy when we are linked to a source of meaning—God—and when we experience relationships that sustain us, nurture us, and point us to God over and over again."

Dr. Morris is following in the footsteps of John Wesley (1703-91) the founder of Methodism, who was a health reformer and a relentless advocate of both spiritual and physical fitness.

Dr. Morris challenges churches to reclaim this commitment to health and the healing ministry of Jesus. He challenges individual congregations to get involved "by envisioning their role in the health of members and the community around them." He challenges individual Christians to "get involved in changing health care by taking charge of their own health care."

Dr. Morris wrote recently in the *Church Health Reader*:

"The church should be concerned about health care. Why? The simple answer is, of course, because Jesus was. Sick people came to him in droves and he exhausted himself with a healing ministry as much as a preaching ministry.

"The church can be a voice that brings the conversation back to talking about improved health outcomes, rather than how to pay for a broken system.

"In this country we believe that no matter what we do to our bodies, doctors can use technology to fix them when they break, or when we break them. Unfortunately, the technology is not always that good, and the doctor is not always that smart.

"Churches have the potential to be powerhouses of life-giving community by advocating for prevention, and teaching people how to care for both their bodies and their spirits, and live healthy lifestyles.

"Revitalization of the church will not come from bad Christian rock music; but it may indeed come from creative, active, health ministries all over the country."

The Center recently launched a new magazine, *Church Health Reader*, to assist churches nationwide in fostering health education and prevention. More information on the Center is available at www. churchhealthcenter.org.

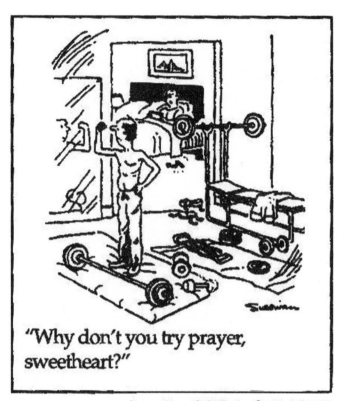

"Why don't you try prayer, sweetheart?"

from *JoyfulNoiseletter.com*
©Ed Sullivan

Chapter 17

The Healing Power of Prayer and Loving Care

The efforts to restore Jesus' healing ministry have taken many forms, especially in the 20th century.

The International Order of St. Luke the Physician, an inter-denominational order dedicated to the Christian helping ministry, was founded in 1932 by Rev. John Gayner Banks, an Episcopal priest. Members of the ecumenical order, belonging to a variety of Christian denominations, pray for the physically or emotionally ill with the laying on of hands. Members of the order—both clergy and laypeople—meet together in several hundred chapters in the U.S. and Canada.

My friend, the late Rev. Canon Alfred W. Price, rector of St. Stephen's Episcopal Church in Philadelphia, was the warden of the Order of St. Luke. Rev. Canon Price invited me to become a member and to attend a healing service in the beautiful old Gothic church. Outside on the front of the church is a plaque declaring: "Built in 1822 on the site where Ben Franklin flew his famous kite."

I've learned that I can always pray for someone when I don't have the strength to help them in some other way.

–Andy Rooney

I participated in the prayers and laying on of hands for the sick at this and other OSL healing services. And I was astonished at the number of sick people who were healed or helped. "But why should you be astonished?" one OSL old-timer asked me. "Prayer is the expression of God's love and caring for all people, and He wishes to bless us."

Rev. Canon Price had a great sense of humor, and he became a consulting editor to *The Joyful Noiseletter.*

Two remarkable women, Agnes Sanford (1897–1982) and Catherine Marshall (1914–1983) were instrumental in sparking a wave of interest in spiritual healing in mainline Christian churches.

Sanford, born in China the daughter of Presbyterian missionaries, was a key figure in the charismatic movement of the 1960's and 1970's and the founder of the Inner Healing Movement. Her book, *The Healing Light*, sold over a half-million copies. The Agnes Sanford Order of St. Luke School of Pastor Care was named in her honor.

Hate and fear can poison the body as surely as any toxic chemicals.

–Joseph Krimsky

Catherine Marshall, whose father was a Presbyterian pastor, married Peter Marshall, the pastor of the New York Avenue Presbyterian Church in Washington, DC in 1936. He also became Chaplain of the United States Senate.

She later wrote a biography of her husband, titled *A Man Called Peter,* and wrote 30 books, including *Adventures in Prayer*, which sold over 16 million copies. Some years ago, Catherine Marshall wrote: "Many preachers have emphasized Christ as 'the man of sorrows' but have almost completely ignored the fact that Jesus loved people, loved to mingle with them, and had a rare sense of humor."

When she was bedridden and despondent for several years with a serious lung ailment, she suddenly awoke one night in total darkness, and sensed a powerful Presence in her room. "Why do you take yourself so seriously?" the Presence asked her. "Relax! There's nothing I can't take care of." The Presence was loving and almost merry, with a teasing, light banter. The encounter was a turning point in her illness and put her on the road to good health.

"The Jesus I had met was oh, so different from the Jesus pictured in most Sunday school books or painted by most artists—solemn, sad-eyed, plodding on His sorrowful way to Cavalry."

Later, Marshall was delighted when the Quaker theologian Dr. Elton Trueblood authored a book titled, *The Humor of Christ.* "One obvious reason why we have not recognized so much of Jesus' humor: we are missing the tone of voice and facial expression," Marshall wrote. "This is a great loss, for much of a person's wit and banter are revealed by his happy expression and personality."

One of the most saintly people I've known is a priest few people have ever heard of: Fr. Peter Mary Rookey, OSM, founder of the International Compassion Ministry, based in Chicago. Fr. Rookey, a Catholic priest in the Order of Friar Servants of Mary for 73 years, was known as "the healing priest" and served all people who sought him or called him seeking prayers, including unbelievers.

Since he co-founded the ministry in 1987, thousands of people with a variety of ailments have come to him seeking prayers for healing. And the ministry's newsletter for years has been filled with witness letters testifying to healings from everything from depression to cancer.

I was blessed to have Fr. Rookey as a friend. He was a humble man with a keen sense of humor who lived simply and occasionally contributed to *The Joyful Noiseletter*. When one of my friends developed a serious illness, I called him in his Chicago office (he usually answered the phone himself) and asked him to pray for him. We prayed together, and in a week's time, my friend made a remarkable recovery.

He was also health-minded and recommended to some of the sick who contacted him that they change their diets.

Before he died, Fr. Rookey expressed his concern that more priests aren't carrying on Jesus' mission of healing. "Priests today are afraid that someone might not get healed," he said.

He died in 2014 at the age of 97.

God uses many different instruments to heal, and one of the most charismatic was the Methodist-Pentecostal televangelist Oral Roberts (1918–2009). Roberts began his ministry as a traveling faith healer in Oklahoma.

He conducted faith healing crusades around the world, praying for, and laying hands on, thousands of sick people who stood in line for him. Many reported healings.

He began his ministry as a member of the Pentecostal Holiness Church, but later became a member of a Methodist church in Tulsa.

Roberts' style was flamboyant, and his televangelism ministry prospered. He was able to raise sufficient funds to build Oral Roberts University.

He was able to buy holiday homes in Palm Springs and Beverly Hills, and three Mercedes cars, and was fond of wearing Italian silk suits, diamond rings, and gold bracelets.

Roberts was criticized for preaching a "Health and Prosperity Gospel," which contrasted with John Wesley's concern for the poor and Wesley's "Health and Poverty Gospel." Whatever his faults, Roberts dramatically focused people's attention on the power of prayer.

He died in 2009 at the age of 91.

Another valuable spiritually-oriented ministry is Stephen Ministries, a lay caregiving ministry that supplements pastoral care. Founded in 1975 by Lutheran Pastor Kenneth C. Haugk, a clinical psychologist, Stephen Ministries trains and teaches laypersons to provide one-on-one care for individuals who request support in congregations.

Reasons for requesting a Stephen minister's visit may range from grieving the loss of a loved one, going through a divorce, experiencing a major illness, job loss, or struggling with substance abuse.

The confidential caregiver and care-receiver relationship, usually conducted by weekly visits, may continue for months or years. (Members of Alcoholics Anonymous long have recognized the value of a "buddy" system.)

Pg. 102

Stephen Ministries' central office is located in St. Louis, Missouri, and more than 12,000 congregations from 160 Christian denominations are now involved in the U.S., Canada, and 24 other countries.

I have participated in healing services, prayers, and the laying on of hands with charismatics from *all* Christian faith traditions: Pentecostals, Assembly of God, Methodists, Lutherans, Episcopalians, Catholics, and Greek Orthodox. And I have been amazed by the spiritual power and healings I've seen and experienced, no matter what the theology of the people who were praying. Proof, perhaps, that it is God alone who heals.

So long as we are in conflict with our body, we cannot find peace of mind.

–George Feuerstein

The healing power of prayer, the healing power of the caring human touch, and the healing power of joyful spiritual music still works miracles.

Some were healed immediately from a variety of ailments. Others were healed over a period of time. Still others experienced healings, but relapsed when they returned to an unhealthy lifestyle. And still others were not healed.

The charismatic movement grew dramatically in many churches during the 1960s, 1970s, and 1980s, but then it declined dramatically at a time when healing ministries were even more greatly needed.

I believe that its decline could be attributed to several factors:

- Its failure to recognize the physiological, nutritional, and environmental factors in the disease process.

- The elitist charismatic leaders who insisted that a sign of the Holy Spirit was "speaking in tongues," and unless the person prayed for spoke in tongues, he or she didn't really have the Holy Spirit.

- Some charismatic leaders and preachers had the deserved reputation of being relentlessly solemn and humorless, forgetting that the fruit (and gift) of the Holy Spirit was joy—and humor and laughter are an expression of that joy. "Blessed are you who weep; you shall laugh." (Luke 6:21) "Be of good cheer, I have overcome the world." (John 16:23) "The One whose throne is in heaven sits laughing." (Psalm 2:4)

- Some of the charismatic leaders became enamored with the alien theories of psychobabble.

Rev. David A. Bullock of Greater St. Matthew Baptist Church in Highland Park, Michigan, organized a prayer vigil in response to the Flint lead-in-water crisis, and had the courage to urge the director of the Michigan Department of Environmental Quality to resign because of it. But many other pastors remained silent on a health issue threatening their congregations.

Rev. Canon Alfred W. Price, warden of the International Order of St. Luke, offered this prayer at the start of a healing service:

> "Our Heavenly Father, we thank You for a saving sense of humor. May we learn to sing through tears and to laugh in spite of sorrow and know that real humor is rooted in an unconquerable faith in the ultimate goodness of God. Help us to laugh at ourselves and not take ourselves too seriously."

Chapter 18

Patch Adams: Clown-Prince of Physicians

Before the movie *Patch Adams* made him famous, Hunter ("Patch") Adams, MD., "the clown-prince of physicians," contributed some wise and wacky articles to the early issues of *The Joyful Noiseletter*.

Patch, a *JN* consulting editor, is a remarkable man with an extraordinary story that the movie told only in part. As a young physician in Washington, D.C., Patch became so deadly serious about everything that he became deeply depressed, tried to kill himself, and committed himself to a mental hospital. There a number of revelations burst into his life.

"I saw how the other patients had alienated their support system—the love—from their lives. There was a recurrent theme of being alone. I grew to respect what matters in life: wonder and curiosity and love and faith and family and friends and nature."

We don't stop playing because we turn old, but turn old because we stop playing.

–Joseph Krimsky

There the real Patch Adams discovered the healing power of faith, humor, and love, and added humor and clowning to his medical practice.

Patch, the clown, now is a popular speaker before medical organizations. He and other health professionals live in community with their patients. He said:

"From the start, "it was obvious to me that we had to have fun in what we were doing. Not only is fun glue

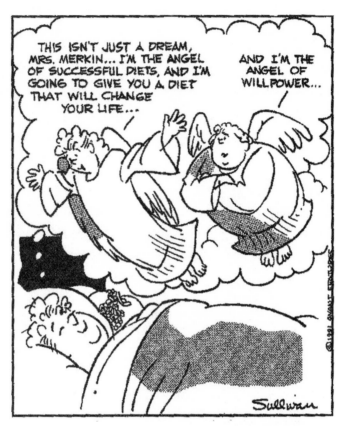

from *JoyfulNoiseletter.com*
©Ed Sullivan

for our community, but it had overwhelming medicinal effects on the patients. So many fewer pain medications! With psychiatric patients, there was overwhelming progress in intimacy and in relieving symptoms.

"After all, what is bedside manner? When you say, 'That doctor has a good bedside manner,' what are you really talking about? The element of love that they bring into the room, and the elements of humor they bring into the room."

Patch is still engaged in his endless campaign to humor and humanize the often chilly world of high-tech medicine.

He believes that humor, laughter, play, celebration, joy, faith, compassion, creativity, and good nutrition are integral parts of the healing process. He has traveled extensively with his clown troupe to 70 countries, including refugee camps, with that message.

Building a Free Clinic

A popular speaker, he has personally raised $1 million in speaker's fees for his organization, the Gesundheit Institute, to realize his dream of establishing the Patch Adams Teaching Center and Clinic in West Virginia.

Patch has enlisted the support of health professionals, including doctors, and nurses, who will live and work at the center, along with their patients, and offer free medical services to patients in one of the poorest rural areas in West Virginia. The teaching center is "a project in holistic medical care," and the clinic's doctors and nurses have committed themselves to work for very modest salaries on 320 acres of land.

"My role models of devoted and caring service were Dr. Albert Schweitzer and Dr. Tom Dooley," Patch wrote in his book, *Gesundheit!* (Healing Art Press). "Faith is the cornerstone of our inner strength, a personal, passionate belief in something of inexhaustible power and mystery... Patients who are full of God need less medication."

Here are some of Patch's thoughts on health and healing:

"One of the most important tenets of our philosophy is that health is based on happiness—from hugging and clowning around to finding joy in family and friends and ecstasy in nature and the arts.

"I insist that humor and fun (which is humor in action) are equal partners with love as key ingredients for a healthy life. Humor forms the foundation of good mental health.

"Many hospitals have realized the importance of faith and have included pastors on the staff. The same could be done with humor: hire clowns and playful people.

"After I gave a 'playshop' at DeKalb Medical Center in Decatur, Georgia, one doctor surveyed the patients the next day to find out whether they'd rather go to a 'goofy' or solemn part of the hospital. Everybody voted for 'the goofy ward.'"

Deadly Serious Psychiatry

"Psychiatry is supposed to be the science of the mind, but I have been unable to find even one paragraph devoted to happiness in a psychiatry textbook. I never hear mental health professionals prescribing happiness to the mentally unhealthy.

"Psychiatric journal ads promoting tranquilizers and 'talk therapies' aim merely at helping patients *cope* with their problems

"When I was a medical student, joylessness prevailed not only on the hospital wards but in the medical classrooms as well. All other facets of the patient's life—family, friends, faith, fun, work, integrity, nutrition, exercise—were considered virtually irrelevant to the medical practice.

"The psychiatry textbooks did not discuss any aspects of a healthy, happy life, much less suggest how to attain it. Instead, they were filled with descriptions of pathology and case histories of bizarre mental disease.

"Getting close to patients was forbidden. There was no friendliness or laughter.

"In psychiatry, the need for professional distance was magnified multifold. Whenever we showed any regard for the patient's pain, we were sharply criticized for 'getting too involved.' God forbid we should have an impulse to touch a patient! I remember how much excitement was generated when some of the staff tried to develop a computer program that could interview the patient, thus eliminating the need for human interaction entirely!

The arrival of a good clown exercises more beneficial influence upon the health of a town than of 20 asses laden with drugs.

–Dr. Thomas Sydenham, 17th-century English physician

"The patient's faith was listed without indicating whether it was an active force in his or her current life. The doctor-as-technician tendency seemed to have gone berserk.

"Bedside manner is the unabashed projection of love, humor, empathy, tenderness, and compassion for the patient."

Perking Up Patients

"The best fun of all was interacting with patients. I rebelled against grand rounds and the impersonality of 10 strangers in white coats trooping into a sick person's room. The air of solemnity was so thick that I preferred to visit patients when the heavies weren't around.

"I discovered that if I entered a hospital room and was vibrant and smiley, the patient would immediately perk up. I discovered that the patients were thrilled to have me there. I was free to talk with the patients, cry with them, massage them, comfort them, joke with them, and inject some exuberance and fun into their lives.

"The patients loved it. The nurses loved it. My fellow medical students were another story.

"Humor is an antidote to all ills. Life is such a miracle and it's so good to be alive that I wonder why anybody ever wastes a minute.

"People crave laughter as if it were an essential amino acid. Health education does little to develop the skills of levity.

"Comic relief is a major way for folks to dissipate pain. One of the best aids in the transition from a 'heavy' to a 'light' existence is to open up the comedian in one-self. People are hungry for humor, so if you can be silly around them, their thanks will garland your life."

"A plague in our society has struck all income levels and social classes, and threatens our future security. No medication can eradicate it, and no vaccine or immunization can prevent it. This plague—the breakdown of the family—is symptomatic of an unhealthy society.

"In more than 30 years as a physician, I never have seen any suffering that begins to touch the horror of loneliness. The cries of this condition are gut-wrenching, and only friendship can really ease the pain... One way to support lonely people is to help them recreate an extended family with friends. And that is what we will do at our hospital."

Patch's free clinic will focus not only on the healing power of humor, play, clowning, and recreation, but also on the health benefits of good nutrition and physical fitness.

"We will use nature to rekindle wonder and curiosity," Patch said. "Whether walking up our mountain, fishing in the lake, or studying with a microscope, patients and staff will find rapture in nature's bosom."

Nature as Physician

"Nature, the attending physician, will help us explore beauty and inspiration. The gardens will have a palette of color, sound, smell, and touch that will melt even the hardest heart. Everybody will have a hand in creating the gardens."

Patch recommends a balanced, nutritious, plant-based diet, and suggests visitors bring fresh-cut fruits and vegetables on platters for hospital patients and staff.

Patch hopes to complete the center in three years. It will provide sleeping, eating, and meeting space for up to 100 visitors. It will house an extensive research library of over 30,000 titles, including all of the editions of *The Joyful Noiseletter* which Patch has received as a subscriber.

A young woman medical doctor in a Kalamazoo, Michigan, hospital observed recently that "some of the old guard in the medical profession scoffed at Patch Adams when the movie came out, but Patch has made a difference with the younger doctors."

The idea for a free hospital may seem bizarre, unless you have read the New Testament and know that Jesus and his disciples healed many of the sick and suffering from a variety of ailments—without charging them a shekel—a major reason for the great popularity of early Christianity among the masses. They did this with faith, love, and good cheer and by encouraging people to change their unhealthy lifestyles.

Additional information on the Patch Adams Teaching Center and Clinic is available from the Gesundheit Institute, 122 Franklin St., Urbana, IL 61801, or from its website—www.PatchAdams.org.

Patch still makes house calls, and in his book *House Calls* (Robert D. Reed Publishers) offers some wise and entertaining advice on "how we can heal the world one visit at a time."

Patch's book, merrily illustrated with cartoons by Jerry Van Amerongen, shows anyone how to visit hospital patients and bring love, humor, compassion, friendship, and hope to promote healing.

In this book, you'll see the real Patch Adams, whom you saw only in part in the movie.

Chapter 19

The Healing Power of Humor

*F*amily *Circus* cartoonist Bil Keane, a consulting editor to *The Joyful Noiseletter*, once remarked: "My friends, humorists Erma Bombeck and Art Buchwald have done far more for the health of humanity than Madame Curie or Dr. Christiaan Barnard."

"Angels can fly because they take themselves lightly," wrote G.K. Chesterton. "Never forget that the devil fell by force of gravity. He/she who has the faith has the fun."

For 30 years, *The Joyful Noiseletter* has received endless examples of the healing power of humor from health professionals, doctors, nurses, counselors, hospital and military chaplains, pastors of all faith traditions, comedians, clowns, and cartoonists.

There was a restaurant in Pittsburgh owned and managed by a high-spirited clown and cut-up named Barney. Barney was beloved, had a host of friends, and when a person entered his restaurant, he would announce their name on a loudspeaker.

One day, one of Barney's friends was eating his dinner at a table when he suddenly clutched his chest, keeled over, and tumbled to the floor, his face ashen. Barney asked a waiter to call an ambulance, rushed to his side, and cradled him in his arms.

Barney whispered in his year: "You're going to be okay, Sam. Have you paid your check?"

The stricken man laughed—and laughed and couldn't stop laughing. The complexion of his face changed from ashen to a healthy ruddy color, and with some help he got to his feet, still laughing, assuring everyone that he felt fine. He was still laughing when he was carried out on a stretcher to the ambulance, bound for the hospital.

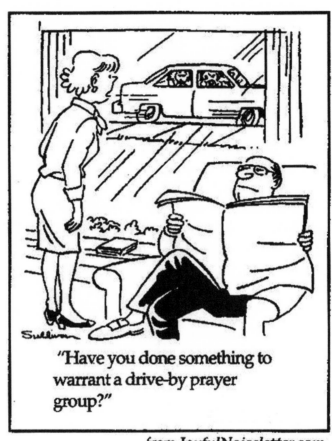

"Have you done something to warrant a drive-by prayer group?"

from *JoyfulNoiseletter.com*
©Ed Sullivan

A young man entered a Minnesota hospital deeply depressed and suicidal. He refused to eat or to talk to anyone or to cooperate with the doctors or nurses. He simply stayed in bed staring at the ceiling.

A nurse who was a clown asked the staff if she could try a different approach. She dressed in a Batman mask and a cloak one day, climbed onto the window sill, and leaped over the young man's bed. That got the young man's attention and broke the ice. Finally, he talked. The nurse told him a few jokes, and amazingly, he started to laugh. Then she talked him into eating his dinner.

He opened up to her, and as she held his hand, told her his troubles. He needed a friend and a caring ear. His depression slowly dissipated. He was discharged and returned to his job a month later.

The Joyful Noiseletter's subscribers include numerous clowns who visit hospitals and nursing homes and whose experiences attest to the healing power of humor. One of our consulting editors, Don (Ski the Clown) Berkoski and his wife, Ruby, founded Smiles Unlimited in Indianapolis, and trained clowns to go into hospitals throughout the state of Indiana and cheer up patients.

The Berkoski's helped teach clowning to the troubled youngsters in the adolescent psychiatric unit at Methodist Hospital in Indianapolis. "I know Ski's program has helped heal some very troubled minds," said Renard Alotta, a hospital therapeutic recreation specialist.

The Catholic Berkoski family put on shows for which they never charged. "Clowns can take away some of the hurt and pain people are going through by giving away hugs and unconditional love—free-of-charge," Ski said.

People with a sense of humor tend to be less egocentric and more realistic in their view of the world and more humble in moments of success and less defeated in times of travail.

–Bob Newhart

Don Berkoski was the first clown ever to receive the Sagamore of the Wabash Award, the highest honor bestowed by the Governor of Indiana, Gov. Evan Bayh, for his efforts to make clowns available to every hospital, nursing home, and prison in the state.

Cleone Lyvonne Reed of Bandon, Oregon, has developed five clown characters of her own and views clowning as "a sacred and spiritual journey" for both believers and nonbelievers.

She is the author of a delightful book on clowning titled *The Sacred Art of Clowning... and Life!* (Robert D. Reed Publishers).

"We can minister to people through caring clowning, such as hospitals and nursing homes, regardless of our religious beliefs," she says. "To be a clown is to be dedicated to a love of life and a life of love."

In Cleone's "Joy of Clowning Playshop," she trained a wheelchair-bound woman with cerebral palsy. The woman took the clown named "Wings" because "I am flying free of my limitations." And she went back to college to work on her master's degree.

Two of Cleone's favorite hospital clowning stories are as follows:

Chloe the Clown Consumes Chocolate Candy

"When I lived in Seattle, I clowned in two different hospitals with a clown who called himself Doc Ouch. He wore a stethoscope around his neck with a toilet plunger on the end.

"One day, we entered a room where a man maybe in his seventies was lying all hooked up to a bunch of tubes. His wife was on one side of the bed and his son maybe in his forties or fifties was on the other side.

"The patient's wife offered me a piece of chocolate. In normal situations, I would have merely said 'no thank you' and gone on with some clown antics of one kind or another. However, the spirit inside of me knew deeply somehow that to refuse this gift would have hurt her feelings. It was a gift to her for me to be able to receive and thus give her the pleasure of giving.

"I enthusiastically accepted a piece of chocolate and ate it very slowly. I savored every bite. I rolled my eyes, closed my eyes, and oohed and aahed with every bite. I chewed each bite exploring every taste bud in my mouth. It was a real performance just to eat this piece of chocolate in slow motion. All eyes were on me the entire time. I commanded their attention with simplicity—silliness of a rather sublime kind.

"When I finished eating the candy, I suddenly turned my eyes towards Doc Ouch and said in a high, innocent quick voice, 'Doc Ouch, do you want to check my heart?'

"He said, 'Suuurrreee. I do.'

"I then faster than you could blink an eye turned my body around, lifted up my can-cans and full skirt revealing my pink bloomers with a big satin heart on my butt, the heart surrounded by fancy lace, and he plopped that stethoscope right on my heart!

"The patient laughed so hard and spontaneously with the surprise of it all that I thought he would fall out of his tubes."

Divine Healing

"This divine energy is also a source of healing. When I did hospital clowning in Seattle, I entered a room one day as Chloe the Clown with a friend, Samarita Perez from Puerto Rico, clown name Payasa (which is clown in Spanish). As I do often, I waved a little stuffed cat toy in front of a patient's chest and asked her what I was doing. (Many people guess I am hypnotizing them. The correct answer is that I am giving them a cat scan!) This very thin frail woman did not care what I was doing.

"She looked into my eyes, and said, 'Did you bring me healing?'

"Payasa heard her and asked very affirmatively, 'Do you want some healing?'

"Payasa held her ankles for a long time while I stood by her bedside and held my hands about a foot or so above her chest and held a prayerful meditative stance. Several of her woman friends were in the room, and everyone held a most sacred space of silence and reverence for quite some time.

"When we left the room, Payasa and Chloe joined Doc Ouch and the three of us held hands and the tears rolled down our faces. Doc Ouch said, 'I don't know what went on in there, but it sure was very powerful.'

"I told this story at a church service in Texas, and a woman came up to me afterwards and said, 'You know, Payasa did that all wrong. She shouldn't have been holding her ankles! She should have been holding her heels.'

"Very puzzled, I looked at her and said, 'Why?'

"She said, 'Because it was a HEELING!'"

Red Skelton was one of Cleone's favorite clowns. Skelton once said:

"I'm nuts and I know it. But so long as I make 'em laugh, they ain't going to lock me up.

"If by chance someday you're not feeling well and you should remember some silly thing I've said or done and it brings back a smile to your face or a chuckle to your heart, then my purpose as your clown has been fulfilled.

"Live by this credo: have a little laugh at life and look around you for happiness instead of sadness. Laughter has always brought me out of unhappy situations.

"No matter what your heartache may be, laughing helps you forget it for a few seconds."

Presbyterian Pastor Bud Frimoth ("Doolotz") and his wife, Lenore ("Wrinkles"), of Portland, Oregon, clowned for decades in hospitals and nursing homes.

They put on workshops on clowning at a camp for sexually abused girls in Oregon, and put smiles back onto their faces. Bud and Lenore gave the girls the confidence they needed to venture out onto the streets as clowns in Astoria. "It's marvelous to see these young girls find ways of expressing themselves through clowning," said Lenore.

Bud chose the name "Doolotz" for his tramp clown name because the Greek word for servant is *doulos* and "a tramp clown is a form of a servant."

A New York foundation announced it has financed a $150,000 study to determine if laughter really is the best medicine. The project sent 35 clowns into New York children's hospitals three times a week to entertain the children.

Another *Joyful Noiseletter* consulting editor, Sr. Mary Christelle Macaluso of Omaha, Nebraska—aka "The Fun Nun"—founded the Order of Fun Nuns, and brought lots of laughter to the academic world.

Comedienne Marlo Thomas, the daughter of Danny Thomas, observed: "The rejection that we all take and the sadness and the aggravation and the loss of jobs and all of the things that we live through in our lives, without a sense of humor, I don't know how people make it."

Chaplain's Humor Opens Self-made Tombs

After serving as pastor of several Baptist churches in North Carolina, Rev. Jack Hinson brought healing humor and laughter to patients as chaplain at Harris Regional Hospital in Sylva, North Carolina, for 14 years. "Chaplain Jack" has written an amazing story about the close cooperation between a joyful, witty chaplain and the medical doctors and nurses at the hospital in his book, *Laughter was God's Idea: Stories about Healing Humor.*

Here are some excerpts from Rev. Hinson's book:

"Joy surprises us and cracks open our self-made tombs to invite us to see the world through God's grace. (And isn't that what Easter is all about?)

"I became the hospital's first full-time chaplain in 1986. After 18 months of walking with individuals through pain, suffering, anger, grief, despair, hopelessness, helplessness, and a whole sea of negativity, I discovered I was becoming overwhelmed.

"A pervasive cloud of doubt, inadequacy, and defeat had invaded my soul. How could a depressed chaplain minister to people in urgent need of healing? I considered resigning.

"Then, at a pastor's conference, I heard Conrad Hyers (a Presbyterian pastor) give a lecture that ultimately reframed my perception of the healing power of humor, joy, and laughter."

"G.K. Chesterton (a Catholic) added to the intrigue when I read what he wrote: 'Pride is the downward drag of all things into an easy solemnity. Seriousness is not a virtue... It is a vice. It is really a natural trend into taking one's self gravely, because it is the easiest thing to do. Solemnity flows out of men naturally; but laughter is a leap. It is easy to be heavy; hard to be light.'

"I discovered that I was taking myself too seriously and not taking God seriously enough. This new insight transformed my ministry at the hospital.

"Now, viewed from my deeper perception of joy, I could face my duties with renewed purpose.

"Joy rises up to produce humility... Joy is a sign of the truly redeemed spirit that gives life its most intense energy. Joy is the work of God's grace within us reminding us of the Christ who said, 'I have spoken this to you so that my joy may be in you and your joy complete.' (John 15:11)

"Joy enables us to let go of the dark and foreboding events that tend to color life in shades of gray. Joy opens up new avenues of courage and confidence, and spills over into a sense of adventure.

"Joy releases us from the need to put ourselves in the center of everything, isolating us from one another. In our seriousness, we become full of seriousness; we become full of ourselves, our anxiety, our agony, our loneliness, and our emptiness. Our joy draws us together to help one another.

"I believed the hospital deserved a joyful chaplain. My prayer was: God, if you will furnish the joy, I will spread it all over the hospital—in every room, in the halls, in the cafeteria, in the chapel, in the lobby, on the grounds. I will deliver a joyful, cheerful spirit.

"Harris Regional Hospital's Pastoral Care Department, in cooperation with western Carolina University and *The Joyful Noiseletter*, sponsored a national conference on 'The Healing Power of Humor' in 1990.

"I discovered that most patients and their families appreciated a cheerful chaplain who could help them forget themselves, if only for a few minutes. So I set about my work with a greater sense of purpose when I adopted God's wonderful gift of healing through humor.

Finding some humor in today's many problems is the next best thing to solving them.

–Tom Mullen

"Good humor, used correctly, can save us from ourselves. It becomes our ally, our friend, our advocate.

"People who cannot laugh at themselves are locked into a jail of seriousness. Fear keeps them in chains. But a little laughter is the key to unlock the prison. And a comic vision helps keep the prison door open forever.

"Maintaining a comic vision will guarantee the realistic perspective for living intended by the Creator. Such a perspective allows people to experience the humorous life in good times and bad.

"Meister Eckhart, the 13th-century mystic, has another gem of wisdom for all who take themselves too seriously: 'God is enjoying Himself and He expects us to join him.'

"Right in the middle of life, where people are willing to take the leap of laughter, amazing miracles happen: blood pressure is leveled, oxygen surges to the brain, and endorphins are produced.

"And you and I have extraordinary opportunities at every point to 'attack' our violent world with the greatest tool on earth—*Love*. Love is needed everywhere. Let it loose anywhere, and it works its way into any situation.

"I once visited a shut-in who made a stunning remark as I hugged her on the way out: 'Pastor, that is the only hug I ever get, and I thank you.'

"I did not understand the importance of human touch until I learned from medical sources that hugging is an excellent tonic, helps lift depression, tunes up the body's immune system, and helps control pain.

"I had different ties that I wore to the hospital. I call them 'bridge ties' because they help me connect with a patient. I have Mickey Mouse, Charlie Chaplin, Three Stooges, Looney Tunes, a Tabasco Shrimp, and a frog tie.

"After 14 years of dosing out daily spoonfuls of healing humor to patients, loved ones, and members of the hospital staff, I'm convinced that laughter is still the best medicine.

"Laughter had an extraordinary impact on my chaplaincy. My prayer is that readers will gain insight and courage to accept God's gift of laughter as a means to enjoy life and make God's world a better place to live by taking excessive doses of laughter every day and by sharing this extraordinary gift with others.

"I urge people not to go into eternity having to give account for all of the laughter you could have enjoyed but did not.

"Laughter was God's idea. Let him bless you with it every day."

Karen Buxman, RN, a contributing editor to *The Journal of Nursing Jocularity,* authored an entertaining book titled *This Won't Hurt a Bit! And Other Fractured Truths in Health Care,* replete with health care humor. "I believe firmly that laughter helps the medicine go down," Buxman wrote. "Humor gives us hope. It gives us relief. And it gives us victory. Laughter is God's hand wiping the tears away from one's heart."

The Chaplain as Will Rogers

Another hospital chaplain, Rev. E.T. (Cy) Eberhart, a United Church of Christ pastor in Salem, Oregon, and a consulting editor to *The Joyful Noiseletter*, researched the life of Will Rogers—America's most beloved humorist and journalist since Mark Twain—and did impersonations of Rogers for churches and civic groups.

Rogers, the biracial Cherokee Indian cowboy from Oklahoma, was so popular that in 1928, *Life* magazine did a spoof nominating him as the presidential candidate for the Anti-Bunk Party. In his acceptance speech, Rogers observed that "both parties have lied to folks for so long" that an Anti-Bunk Party was needed to set things straight. He promised that he would not solicit funds from anyone and would resign if elected.

Rogers was raised a Methodist, but when he died his memorial service was presided over by a Protestant minister, a Catholic priest, and a Yiddish performer singing a Hebrew mourning chant. Over 100,000 mourners walked past his casket.

Typical of Rogers' humor was this commentary:

"If there are people who think they come from a monkey, it's not our business to rob them of what little pleasure they may get out of imagining it. What good will it do at this late date to argue over who we came from? The Lord didn't leave any room for doubt when He told you how you should act when you got here. His example and the Ten Commandments are plain enough. So let's just start from there."

"People of all parties and beliefs saw Rogers as one of their own," Rev. Eberhart said. "He radiated hope and humor and joy in the darkest times of the Great Depression."

The late humorist Grady Nutt, a Baptist pastor, said of Will Rogers: "He (Jesus) makes the most sense to me, the most profound impact on me, when I envision him as Will Rogers in sandals."

Exercise Your Funny Bone

Cheryl Bee Fell, R.N. (aka "Nurse Funshine") of Scott, Louisiana, urges patients to "exercise your funny bone" and makes these observations about the healing power of laughter:

Laughter is the cheapest form of over-the-counter medicine... it doesn't cost a penny.

Laughter doesn't require a prescription, a referral from your primary physician nor precertification from your HMO, PPO, or CEO.

Laughter is an old-fashioned remedy that is still recommended today.

Laughter is like a miracle drug without side-effects. There is one warning: laughter may cause a temporary "on-the-edge" hangover.

Laughter does not require batteries... one heartfelt laugh will recharge your funny bone for hours.

Laughter is the best kept dieting secret because silliness is soul food with *zero* calories.

Laughter gives one a shot of energy and a transfusion of hope.

Laughter is like internal jogging... 20 seconds of genuine laughter is equal to approximately 3 minutes of rowing.

John D. Romm, M.D., a Beverly Hills, California physician, passed on this item from the *Mayo Clinic Health Letter*:

"It's been said that laughter is the best medicine. While that's not true for every ailment, research is slowly validating what many people intuitively experience while watching a comedy, having a gab session with funny friends or hearing a well-placed one-liner—that laughter is often an important component of health and well-being for yourself and those around you.

"If it's been a while since you've had a good long belly laugh, you may want to consider taking steps to bring laughter and humor—and its health benefits—into your life."

Prof. Don L.F. Nilsen of Tempe, Arizona, executive secretary of the International Society for Humor Studies, wrote: "Albert Schweitzer was a medical doctor who employed humor not only to combat depression but also to keep from falling into a state of helplessness."

Writing in *Lutheran Libraries*, church librarian Mary Margaret Jordan of Newton, Iowa, said that "humor and hypochondria" are natural enemies, and urged church librarians to include religious humor in their libraries.

Dr. Schweitzer always collected an amusing story or two during the day to share with the young doctors and nurses during mealtimes at Schweitzer Hospital in Africa.

Humor as a Survival Tool for Minorities

Another *Joyful Noiseletter* consulting editor, Rev. Dr. O. Wendell Davis, pastor of Union Chapel Missionary Baptist Church in Huntsville, Alabama, observes that a great deal of joy and humor is expressed in African-American churches.

Dr. Davis writes and delivers his sermons seriously and passionately, but when he stands in the pulpit on Sunday, seriousness often gives way to moments of laughter, and his congregation loves it.

Dr. Davis wrote his Ph.D. dissertation on the history and growth of African-American churches.

"In one of the greatest of the historical ironies, the majority of slaves—owned mainly by white Christian masters—converted to Christianity during 'The Great Awakening' from the early 1800's to 1850," he said.

He observed that many of the slaves developed a keen sense of humor, and that their Christian faith and sense of humor were survival tools under the most dreadful of circumstances. This keen sense of humor was passed on from generation to generation, he said.

The African-American evangelist Marshall Keeble, the son of two former slaves, was famous for his wit and sense of humor, and had both whites and blacks rollin' in the aisles.

When he read German philosopher Friedrich Nietzsche's declaration "God is dead," Keeble commented: "I didn't even know He was sick, and I talked to Him this morning."

When Keeble was informed that a fellow preacher had been awarded a Doctor of Divinity degree, Keeble responded that he did not even know that the "Divine" had been ill, but if He was, he reckoned that having a Doctor of Divinity handy would be useful.

Typical of African-American joy and sense of humor was Ernie Banks, the Hall of Fame slugger, who for 19 years maintained his infectious smile, joyous outlook, nonstop good humor, and boundless enthusiasm for baseball despite decades of playing on miserable Chicago Cub teams who never made the postseason.

As a youngster, Banks played softball for his church's team, and his mother wanted him to follow his grandfather's career as a minister. But he went on to play for a Negro League team before his contract was purchased by the Cubs.

He hit 512 home runs for a perennially losing team but he always reflected optimism. They called him "Mr. Cub" and "Mr. Sunshine," and all of Chicago mourned when he died at the age of 83.

He was a very kind-hearted and approachable man—a class act and a role model for all ballplayers.

Humor and Health Hangouts (aka 3-H Clubs)

Several pastors associated with *The Joyful Noiseletter* introduced to their churches "Humor and Health Hangouts" for people to meet monthly and share their humor and laughter. The clubs, which meet in churches or homes, have a holistic approach to health with a focus on prevention and helping people to strive to be both spiritually and physically fit.

Enthusiastic groups met at First Methodist Church in Glassboro, New Jersey, started by Rev. Dr. Karl R. Kraft, and at the Church of Good Shepherd in Grafton, West Virginia, a group started by Rev. Dr. Bert Coffman.

The groups stressed that healing humor is just one part—an important part—of a healthy lifestyle, which includes good nutrition, regular exercise, and the stewardship of the body, prayer, and regular worship.

Every meeting was begun with "The Clown's Prayer" of Smiles Unlimited.

The *Joyful Noiseletter's* Holy Humor Sunday celebrations were used as models for the 3-H Club meetings. (see www.joyfulnoiseletter.com)

All Religions Have Valued Humor and Laughter

All religions have valued humor and laughter. The word "laugh" appears for the first time in the Old Testament very early on, in Genesis 17:17. God informs the 100-year-old Abraham that his 90-year-old wife, Sarah, will give birth to a son.

Recognizing a divine sense of humor, Abraham laughed. God commanded Abraham to name his son "Isaac," which in Hebrew means "God's laugh." In Arabic, "Ithaac" also means "he laughs."

After she gave birth to Isaac, it was Sarah's turn to laugh. "Then Sarah said, 'God has given me cause to laugh; all those who hear of it will laugh with me." (Genesis 21:6)

> *Laughter, indeed, is God's therapy.*
>
> –Malcolm Muggeridge

Psalm 2-4 declares: "The One whose throne is in heaven sits laughing." Proverbs 17:22 declares: "A cheerful heart is a good medicine, but a downcast spirit dries up the bones."

In his book, *The Teacher*, Zvi Kolitz tells this story taken from the Talmud: Rabbi Beroka used to visit the marketplace, where the Prophet Elijah appeared to some saintly men to offer them spiritual guidance. Once Rabbi Beroka asked the prophet, "Is there anyone here who has a share in the world to come?"

"No," the prophet replied.

While they were talking, two men passed them by. On seeing them, the prophet remarked, "These two men have a share in the world to come."

Rabbi Beroka then approached and asked them, "Can you tell me what is your occupation?

"We are jesters," they replied. "When we see men depressed, we cheer them up."

I noted the similarity of this story to one of the sayings of Islam's prophet Muhammad in one of the translations of his traditions, which was passed on by Peggy Schreur of Kalamazoo,

Michigan: "He who cheers up a person in difficulties, Allah will cheer him in this world and the next."

That saying is almost as overlooked as Sura 5:32 in the Koran: "If anyone kills a person, it would be as if he killed all mankind. And if anyone saves a life, it would be as if he saved the life of all mankind."

Many of the statutes of Buddha portray him with a smile on his face.

There are numerous references to joy and laughter in the New Testament.

"Happy are you who weep now; you shall laugh," Jesus tells his disciples. (Luke 6:21) And "When you fast, do not put on a gloomy look as the hypocrites do." (Matthew 6:16)

And on the eve of his crucifixion, Jesus tells his disciples: "These things I have spoken to you, that My joy may be in you, and that your joy may be full." (John 15:11)

Christianity recognizes joy as one of the fruits of the Holy Spirit. Humor and laughter are expressions of joy, and it is difficult to understand why so many super-serious theologians have failed to recognize that these, too, are gifts of the Holy Spirit with great healing power.

Chapter 20

The Longevity of Comedians, Humorists, and Clowns

The beloved comedians I remember growing up were, as a rule, a hardy and long-lived breed. Laughter may well be the best medicine.

Bob Hope and George Burns lived to 100. Red Buttons, who lived to 87, credited his longevity to "humor and health foods."

"Eighty is not old," he told the *Journal of Longevity*. "Old is when your doctor no longer X-rays you; he just holds you up to the light. That's old. Old is when you order a two-minute egg and they ask you to pay in advance."

Button stayed physically and mentally active and was keenly aware of the importance of proper nutrition.

"Comedy's a great game to be in for health," he said. "Laughter is a panacea for an awful lot of stuff... Why live a life of road rage?"

Buttons, who was devoted to his synagogue, was a popular speaker at televised special dinners at which he roasted celebrities. He would tell of prominent historical figures who never got a special dinner, like Paul Revere's wife, who said, "I don't care who's coming. It's my night to use the horse."

One of the *Joyful Noiseletter's* consulting editors, Alabama Lutheran Pastor Denny J. Brake, himself an author of several joke books, was inspired by Buttons to put together a list of a few Biblical figures who never got a special dinner:

- Eve, who said to Adam as they were leaving the garden, "Well, dear, we still have each other," didn't get a dinner.

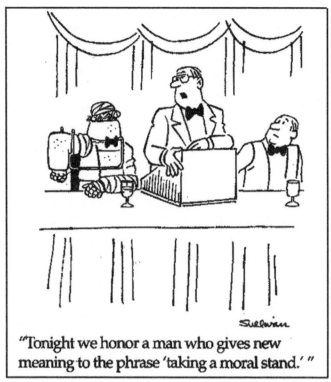

"Tonight we honor a man who gives new meaning to the phrase 'taking a moral stand.'"

from *JoyfulNoiseletter.com*
©Ed Sullivan

- Abraham, who after he learned he would be a father at age 100, asked "Is this covered by Medicare?" didn't get a dinner.

- Moses, who stood at the Red Sea and asked, "Where's the bridge?" didn't get a dinner.

- Joshua, who put posters on the walls of Jericho saying, "Watch for falling rocks," didn't get a dinner.

Here is a list of some long-lived comedians and humorists and their ages:

- Steve Allen (December 26, 1921–October 30, 2000) (78)
- Woody Allen (December 1, 1935–) (80)
- Lucille Ball (August 6, 1911–April 26, 1989) (77)
- Ernie Banks (January 31, 1931–January 23, 2015) (6 days shy of 84)
- Jack Benny (February 14, 1894–December 26, 1974) (80)
- Milton Berle (July 12, 1908–March 27, 2002) (93)
- Victor Borge (January 3, 1909–December 23, 2000) (91)
- Art Buchwald (October 20, 1925–January 17, 2007) (81)
- Carol Burnett (April 26, 1933–) (82)
- George Burns (January 20, 1896–March 9, 1996) (100)
- Red Buttons (February 5, 1919–July 13, 2006) (87)
- Johnny Carson (October 23, 1925–January 23, 2005) (79)
- Sid Caesar (September 8, 1922–February 12, 2014) (91)
- Charlie Chaplin (April 16, 1889–December 25, 1977) (88)
- Tim Conway (December 15, 1933–) (82)
- Jimmy Durante (February 10, 1893–January 29, 1980) (12 days shy of 87)
- Bob Hope (May 29, 1903–July 27, 2003) (100)

- Jerry Lewis (March 16, 1926–) (80)

- Groucho Marx (October 2, 1890–August 18, 1977) (86)

- Jackie Mason (June 9, 1931–) (84)

- Bob Newhart (September 5, 1929–) (86)

- Satchel Paige (July 7, 1906–June 8, 1982) (a month shy of 76)

- Martha Raye (August 27, 1916–October 19, 1994) (78)

- Jim Reed (June 27, 1915–February 9, 2010) (94)

- Andy Rooney (January 14, 1919–November 4, 2011) (92)

- George Bernard Shaw (July 26, 1856–November 2, 1950) (94)

- Red Skelton (July 18, 1913–September 17, 1997) (84)

- Jerry Stiller (June 8, 1927–) (88)

- Danny Thomas (January 6, 1912–February 6, 1991) (79)

- Marlo Thomas (November 21, 1937–) (78)

- Mark Twain (November 30, 1835–April 21, 1910) (74)

- Dick Van Dyke (December 13, 1925–) (90)

- Rev. Dr. Sherwood Eliot Wirt (March 12, 1911–November 8, 2008) (97)

- Henny Youngman (March 16, 1906–February 24, 1998) (3 weeks shy of 92)

Some of these comedians are still alive.

Some of these comedians and humorists continued to play tennis or golf into their senior years. Charlie Chaplin and Groucho Marx were avid tennis players, and were court jesters who had the edge of keeping their opponents in stitches.

If you watch the older movies, you'll observe that, as a rule, most of the comedians of the 1910s, 1920s, and 1930s, were lean, physically fit, and athletic. Charlie Chaplin, Buster Keaton, Harold Lloyd, Groucho Marx, and Red Skelton delighted audiences with their vaudevillian acrobatics.

Many of these comedians took care of themselves, and their lifestyles were healthier. They avoided drugs. All of them retained a humorous and positive attitude towards life.

Many of them were devout Christians, or devout Jews, or at the very least, respectful of religious values. They might be rightly described as the "clean comedians." They were lovable.

Milton Berle would tell the story of the time he went to a hospital to visit his friend, comedian Jim Backus, who had fallen ill. Berle made a great effort to cheer up his friend, and told him his best jokes for an hour. As Berle was leaving, he turned to Backus and said, "I hope you're better."

"You, too," Backus replied.

Cheetah, Tarzan's comic-relief sidekick in the jungle movies of the 1930s, lived to the age of 80.

Cheetah outlived Tarzan (Johnny Weissmuller, an Olympic athlete). The zookeeper in Palm Harbor, Florida, where he spent his final days said the chimp loved "to see people laugh." If Cheetah could talk, he probably would have attributed his longevity to all those bananas, laughs, and climbing trees.

The multi-talented Steve Allen was another lovable comedian. When he was hospitalized with an illness in 1986, he told a reporter his condition was critical: "critical of nurses, critical of doctors, critical of the food, critical of the prices."

Steve Allen was a consulting editor to *The Joyful Noiseletter* and occasionally contributed a joke or an article.

In his final appearance on television in 2001, Allen was interviewed on a panel of comedians on CNBC. He pointedly contrasted contemporary comedians who unmercifully savage politicians and other people, with Will Rogers, who made hilarious comments about politicians but who was universally loved by all the parties.

"There aren't many comedians who are loved today," Allen observed.

He sometimes described himself as an agnostic, but on other occasions, spoke reverently of the mystery of God, lectured on the seven deadly sins, and denounced the immorality of much of present-day television with the zeal of an Old Testament prophet.

He and his wife of 46 years, actress Jane Meadows, contributed generously to the Los Angeles Mission, where they helped dish up dinners for the homeless on Thanksgiving. And when he died, Allen's family requested that a donation be made to his favorite charities: the Salvation Army in Los Angeles and the Los Angeles Mission.

In his last years, Allen led a national campaign on behalf of clean comedy. Allen's national newspaper ad campaign to clean up television programming generated 506,000 letters of support and more than $4.8 million in donations to buy more ads.

The Parents Television Council has run 1,048 full-page ads in 375 newspapers with a photo of Allen and his message:

> "Parents... grandparents... families. TV is leading children down a moral sewer. Are you as disgusted as I am at the filth, vulgarity, sex, and violence TV is sending into our homes? Are you fed up with steamy unmarried sex situations, filthy jokes, perversion, vulgarity, foul language, violence, killings, etc?
>
> "Are you as outraged as I am at how TV is undermining the morals of children... encouraging them to have pre-marital sex... encouraging lack of respect for authority... and shaping our country down to the lowest standards of decency?
>
> "Well now you and I can end it. We can do it by reaching the TV sponsors whose ad dollars make it possible."

Allen reported that the crusade had broad support across the religious and political spectrum. He said he had received letters of support from conservatives and liberals, Christians, Jews, Muslims, atheists, and agnostics.

Allen wrote: "The element of humor is necessary to human beings, necessary for the maintenance of sanity."

But only clean humor is healing. Still, not much has changed on TV since Allen wrote those words.

When an aging Groucho Marx appeared as a guest on the Dick Cavett show, he commented that he didn't go anymore to the comedy clubs where foul-mouthed comedians performed. Said Groucho: "You don't have to be filthy to be funny."

Another remarkable, long-lived humorist who was a consulting editor to *The Joyful Noiseletter* from its earliest years was Msgr. Arthur Tonne. Tonne loved a good joke and collected them for years, filling nine volumes of *Jokes Priests Can Tell*.

Tonne was the gentle and beloved pastor of St. John Neponucene Catholic Church in Pilsen, Kansas, for many years. "I'd never preach without telling a joke," he said. And he held his own when he appeared as a guest on the David Letterman Television Show.

> **"**
> *Everything is changing. People are taking their comedians seriously and the politicians as a joke.*
>
> –Will Rogers

Tonne said he had lived a long life because "I laughed a lot, did pushups along with my morning prayers, ate a lot of fresh fruit, and stayed physically active and lean." In July, when the mulberry trees were bearing fruit, he would take a couple of bed sheets, lay them under a tree, climb the tree, and shake the branches until the mulberries rained down.

Tonne was a relentless peacemaker. He called *The Joyful Noiseletter* "an ecumenical miracle, bringing together in good humor and camaraderie people who ordinarily don't talk to one another." (He lived to the age of 99.)

Another *Joyful Noiseletter* consulting editor and friend, Sherwood Eliot ("Woody") Wirt, a longtime associate and biographer of Billy Graham, authored—at the age of 88—a bestselling book—*Jesus: Man of Joy* (Harvest House).

Rev. Dr. Wirt, a pastor who was the founding editor of *Decision Magazine*, remained very physically and socially active until he went to the Lord at age 97. He swam laps regularly in a pool in Poway, California.

Still another good friend and consulting editor to *The Joyful Noiseletter*, Jim Reed of Cotter, Arkansas, was one of America's great humorists in the down-home tradition of Will Rogers, but he was unsung because he lived modestly and simply. A Methodist layman, Reed served as editor of *The Topeka Daily Capital* in Kansas and later as the first editor of *American Medical News*, the first newspaper of the American Medical Association.

He wrote books titled *The Funny Side of Fishing* and *The Funny Side of Golf*, and he tickled readers with his hilarious collection of Ozark and political humor. He lived a full life to the age of 94.

Send in the Clowns

Many churches throughout the land have revived an old Greek Christian custom of an ongoing celebration of Jesus' resurrection on the Sunday after Easter—"Bright Sunday"—observing "God's last laugh on the devil when He raised Jesus from the dead." The early Greek Christians celebrated with picnics, parties, singing, dancing, joke-telling, and practical jokes on the clergy.

Modern churches have renamed "Bright Sunday" "Holy Humor Sunday," and the ingenious ways they celebrate this special day can be found at www.joyfulnoiseletter.com.

In the retirement community of Penney Farms, FL, a clown troupe called "The Penney Clowns"—all of them in their eighties—celebrate Holy Humor Sunday on the Sunday after Easter every year. One recent Holy Humor Sunday program was called "Jesus is the Life of the Party," and the clowns entered and led the audience in the singing of "Joy, Joy, Joy." There were skits and the telling of "holy humor jokes." Everyone was given a kazoo and asked to play "When the Saints Go Marching In."

The local newspaper, the *Clay County Leader* reported that the hall rang with laughter.

Everyone participated in this closing prayer:

"Lord, grant me a joyful heart and a holy sense of humor. Please give me the gift of faith, to be renewed and shared with others each day. Teach me to love this moment only, looking neither to the past with regret, nor to the future with apprehension. Let love be my guide, and my life a prayer."

Leader: "Go in laughter, go in grace, keep the Lord in your heart and a smile on your face."

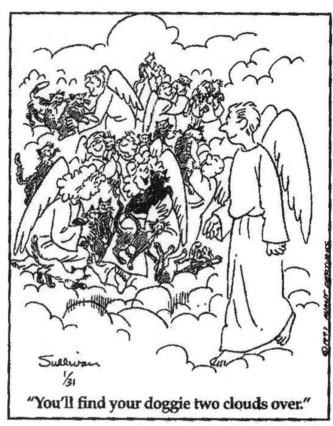

"You'll find your doggie two clouds over."

from *JoyfulNoiseletter.com*
©Ed Sullivan

Chapter 21

The Healing Power of Pets

In the summer of 2014, our 13-year-old Golden Retriever, Maize, became extremely ill, and our vet advised us that it would be merciful to put him down. Driving back home from the vet's office, I—like others who have lost their pets—wept profusely.

Ever since he was a puppy, Maize was a very gentle, sweet-tempered dog who loved everyone. Everybody in our neighborhood—children and adults—loved him and would stop and pet him when we went on walks.

Dogs believe they are human. Cats believe they're God.

–Author unknown

He was a playful and endlessly joyful dog with a steady focus on the present, happy to be alive. He was welcoming to anyone who came into our home, with a wagging tail and a tongue lick to the hand, his way of offering a kiss. He lifted the spirits of anyone who came in contact with him, and made them smile.

When we adopted a cat, he was welcoming and gently playful with her, too. He never snarled at anyone or bit anyone, human or beast. He rarely barked, and never in anger. His occasional barks were invitations to passing dogs to come by and play. If you accidentally stepped on his paw, he would yelp in pain, but he wouldn't retaliate with a bite. He was endlessly forgiving and didn't hold grudges.

When a family member was sick or injured or sad, he would sense their hurt and stay by their side, giving them an occasional hand lick.

During my morning devotions, he would sit patiently at my feet, and after my prayers he would invariably rise and lick my hand.

I thank God for the blessing of Maize's companionship for 13 years. Now that he's gone, I can't help wondering what a better world it would be if more people had Maize's loving, loyal, compassionate, forgiving, uncomplaining, playful and peaceful spirit. I don't pretend to know for sure if pets, when they die, are allowed in heaven. But I believe in a just God, and sometimes I think Maize is more deserving of heaven than I am. I hope to see him again. How can we say goodbye except to say "Well done, good and faithful servant?"

Do Pets Go to Heaven?

When my article about Maize—"A grief observed"—appeared in *The Joyful Noiseletter*, we received many letters from subscribers extolling the virtues of their pets. Here are some of them:

"When I read Cal Samra's article about the death of his Golden Retriever, 'Maize,' I was drawn to tears. I just had to put down my Sheltie of 12 years, 'Harry Potter,' and I am still fighting back tears as I write.

"You did Maize a great honor with your article. He, along with our Harry, was so loving and compassionate.

"I, along with you, thank God for the blessing of our pets.

"I asked my pastor if we would see our pets in heaven when we get there, and he said, 'Anything is possible with God.' I know we shall see Maize and Harry again."

–Jesse Engle, Everett, Pennsylvania

"We received our copy of the Nov.– Dec. *JN* on the day after we had to put to rest our 13-year-old Golden Retriever, Bailey. I have not had the words to express just how much this wonderful animal has meant to my family, but Cal Samra's remembrance of his Golden, Maize, was like seeing my words in print.

"I couldn't believe the timing of this *JN*. Coincidence or divine intervention, your beautiful tribute to your Maize brought me peace. Some of my grief has been replaced with wonder at the creation of these precious and loving spirits. I also thank God for the 13 years we had with Bailey."

–Janet Henry, Plano, Texas

"Cal Samra's article was eloquent and deeply touching. Last winter, we said farewell to our noble, 15-year-old Husky Retriever, Barley. The sight of Barley's trusting eyes, gazing into mine, and then losing focus at the end, is something I shall never forget.

"A week later, we acquired Bella, a 12-year-old Cocker/Chow who had been dumped in a 'kill' shelter. She is a delight. We can say things to pets we would never say to humans, including ourselves. Another blessing of God, and a great one."

–Andy Fisher, Denville, New Jersey

"Cal Samra's article on the passing of his dog was very moving. I draw your attention to Psalm 36.6c: 'You save humans and animals alike, O Lord.' Many pet owners have found comfort in that little verse.

"And why not? If humans were created a little lower than the angels, why shouldn't the animals have been created a little lower than us? And if loyalty, comfort, companionship, and being a source of joy and laughter count for anything, they would certainly be able to add an abundant amount to the heavenly experience."

–Rev. Dr. Karl R. Kraft, Dover, Delaware

"Years ago I had my lab mix, Beau, put down at age 14. I was desperately sad and, in prayer, asked the Lord if I would see my furry friend again.

"A Bible verse came to me. God asked, 'Is anything too difficult for Me?' I considered that a sufficient answer and felt much better.

"A friend at work asked me if I thought there were animals in heaven. I answered: Let's see. You have lambs lying down with wolves, lions eating straw... sounds like animals to me!"

–Allan Stackhouse, Williamsburg, Virginia

Marnelle Thomsen of Virginia Beach, Virginia, passed on a "Prayer at the death of a pet," by Arch Stanton, which reads in part:

"Lord God, my heart is heavy as I face the loss in death of my beloved pet, who was so much a part of my life.

"This pet made my life more enjoyable and gave me cause to laugh and to find joy in his company.

"I remember the fidelity and loyalty of this pet and will miss his being with me. From him I learned many lessons, such as the quality of naturalness and the unembarrassed request of affection.

"In caring for his daily needs, I was taken up and out of my own self-needs, and thus learned to service another.

"May my pet sleep on in an eternal slumber in your Godly care, as all creation awaits the fullness of liberation. Amen."

Dr. Jane R. Westerfield of Dunedin, FL reported that she is the author of a children's book titled, *The Preacher's Dog Goes to Heaven*. The story is told in "First Dog" by a Methodist bishop's Boxer, named "Moreover." The bishop named him for the only dog in the Bible, mentioned in Luke 16:21.

Moreover became the beloved companion of the bishop until the bishop died. Moreover was heartbroken, and when later the dog dies, he is reunited in heaven with the bishop.

Msgr. Robert Ritchie, rector of St. Patrick's Cathedral in New York, was also heartbroken when his beloved yellow Lab "Lexington" died. Lexington was "always full of love since he was a puppy, licking my hand," Msgr. Ritchie said.

When he was in Italy, Ritchie asked an Italian art studio, which carved figures of Jesus, Mary, Joseph and animals for Christmas Nativity scenes, to carve a 25-inch figure of his dog. At the cathedral's annual Christmas concert, some visitors were surprised to see the statue of a dog in the Nativity scene.

One parishioner commented: "I think it makes sense. Jesus was a kind-hearted person, so why wouldn't he have grown up with a dog?"

Charles Daudert reported in his book on Martin Luther's *Table Talks*:

> "When Martin Luther was asked whether dogs and other animals would be in heaven, he answers: 'Yes, certainly... because Peter (Act 3:21) described Judgment Day as a day of restitution of all things, and heaven and earth will be created anew. God will create a new earthly kingdom and heaven (2 Peter 3:13) and will also create a new Tolpel (Luther's dog 'Blockhead')."

For about 20 years, we watched an old man with a U.S. Navy cap shuffle past our house with his small dog on a leash. Over that time we watched him walking three different little mutts. When one dog died, he'd quickly replace it with another. He'd walk his dogs two or three times a day.

I would stop and chat with him occasionally. He said he was 90 years old, and had served on a destroyer in the U.S. Navy during World War II. He was a devout man, with a keen sense of humor, and said he had survived several kamikaze attacks and three marriages. He said that his three dogs had given him more love and laughs than his three wives.

When one day he didn't walk by with his dog, I read in his obituary that he had gone to his eternal rest. I missed him.

"Speed Bump" cartoonist Dave Coverly, a *Joyful Noiseletter* contributing cartoonist, has a new book titled *Dogs Are People, too*. "My family has had two dogs, both rescues, and they've added immeasurably to our live," Coverly said.

A year after my golden retriever Maize died, our family was blessed with another marvelous dog, this one a female lab-mix who came to us by way of the local animal rescue. She had been a stray, brought up from Kentucky; but she was very gentle, loving, and playful.

One of the women at the Kalamazoo Animal Rescue had named her "Bliss," because she seemed so happy and playful. Ironically, she was all white with the exception of a black ring around her left eye. She reminded people of the little white dog with the black ring around his eye in the old "Our Gang" movies. She made you laugh.

Bliss quickly filled the emptiness we had felt after the loss of Maize.

Dog Owners Live Longer

"Dog owners are likely to live longer than other people," according to Jim Reed, first editor of *American Medical News*.

> "The reason is threefold: Since the dog must be taken out for exercise, the exercise the owner himself gets contributes to health and a longer life.
>
> "Two, by giving time and attention to his dog's well-being the owner takes his mind off his own worries, and such contentment is highly beneficial to mental and physical health.
>
> "And three, the dog's ability to act as guard, companion, and friend (particularly to persons living alone) serves to prevent nervousness and encourages relaxation."

Chapter 22

What This Country Needs Is a Good Siesta

From time to time for three decades, *The Joyful Noiseletter* has reported on the health benefits of regular naps and siestas. A study by the Harvard School of Public Health found that a regular afternoon nap could reduce the risk of cardiac death by 37%.

The study followed the lifestyles of 23,681 Greek men and women for three years. Workers who napped regularly, for at least 30 minutes a day, at least three times a week, had the greatest health benefits. Their risk of cardiac death was 64% lower than for those who did not nap.

In Greece, as in other Mediterranean countries, businesses often close shop in mid-afternoon and most people go home and take a siesta. The siesta, the study reported, renews their energy and gives people a healthier heart.

Other studies have shown that many Americans are chronically sleep-deprived and sleep disorders are epidemic.

You will always stay young if you get plenty of rest, eat a balanced diet, exercise moderately, and lie about your age.

–Jim Reed

Dr. Mary A. Carskadon, a professor of psychiatry at Brown University, reported that sleep deprivation and the absence of a midday siesta is seriously affecting the productivity of American students.

On any given day, almost 750,000 American high school students and 100,000 middle-schoolers fall asleep during the school day, Dr. Carskadon told a conference hosted by the National Sleep Foundation.

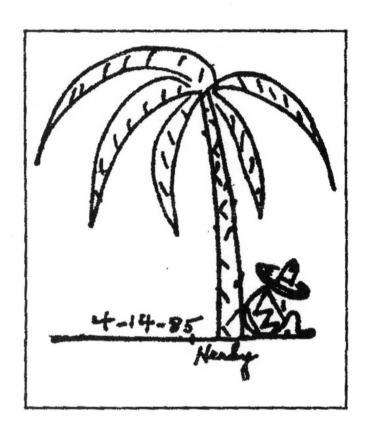

Dr. Carskadon said schools have failed by requiring students to rise too early in the morning to go to school, and by not providing for a midday nap. "It doesn't make sense," she said.

In one school in the Phoenix area located in a Hispanic community, children of Hispanic families who lived near the school were allowed to go home for lunch and a siesta. A teacher at that school told me that the Hispanic children were more energetic and more alert to their studies than the non-Hispanic children who grew tired and less attentive to their studies as the afternoon wore on.

> *A good laugh and a long sleep are the two best cures for anything.*
>
> –Irish Proverb

A lot of schools also have eliminated the daily physical play in gym classes that once were an important part of all schools.

When you deprive children of nap time and physical play time, and feed them on processed foods, fast foods, and junk foods, it should be obvious that you would be fostering a host of behavioral problems and health problems with ailments that only adults got at one time. You don't need a multi-million-dollar study to prove that. All you have to do is read your daily newspaper and watch your local TV news.

Our role models are often the hard-driving, stress-filled, hard-drinking workaholics who have had great success in the business world, but whose lifestyles often wreck their health and put them in early graves.

Check your local newspaper. Not a week goes by without a columnist or editorial writer or pastor eulogizing an "achiever" beloved by his/her family and friends for their "fiercely competitive" qualities and their "tireless" work on their job and on behalf of this or that cause. Gone to the Lord at the tender age of 41 or 47 or 53 or 64, etc.

Here is an excerpt from the obituary of a church leader who tragically died at the age of 48: "He will be long remembered for his 20-hour workdays, his late-night phone calls to his colleagues, and his burning bright desire to spread the Gospel of Jesus Christ through the printed word."

I would venture to suggest that the American business lunch has killed off more people than all the wars of this century. Conducting business over lunch is a sure way to indigestion.

A siesta after lunch relaxes and renews you, and is good for the digestion.

Winston Churchill was a great advocate for the siesta. He always took a nap after lunch, even during the darkest days of World War II. He said it renewed him and enabled him to work late into the night during critical days of the war.

When Jesus slipped away from the crush of the crowds, I believe he did so not only to pray, but also to take a nap.

What does it profit a man to gain the whole world and lose his health?

Chapter 23

The Joyful Noiseletter's Favorite Jokes

About *The Joyful Noiseletter*

For over 30 years, *The Joyful Noiseletter* has been providing jokes pastors can tell in sermons and local church publications. Thousands of subscribers of all faith traditions have sent us the jokes and anecdotes.

A recent United Methodist Church survey found that pastors who bring a sense of humor to the pulpit are the most endearing to their congregations.

Joyful Noiseletter consulting editor Patch Adams, M.D., wrote the following commentary on the occasion of JN's 30th anniversary in 2015:

> "*The Joyful Noiseletter* was launched 30 years ago after the editors visited a seminary library and could not find the word 'humor' in the book index.
>
> "*JN* has filled the sanctuaries and fellowship halls of thousands of churches of all faith traditions with healing laughter.
>
> "Hundreds of humorists, comedians, and clowns, including Steve Allen, Joe Garagiola, George and Peggy Goldtrap, Malcolm Muggeridge, and Rev. Susan Sparks have contributed freely to *JN*.
>
> "Eighteen of America's foremost cartoonists, including Bil and Jeff Keane of 'The Family Circus,' Johnny Hart of 'B.C.,' Dave Coverly of 'Speed Bump,' Ed Sullivan,

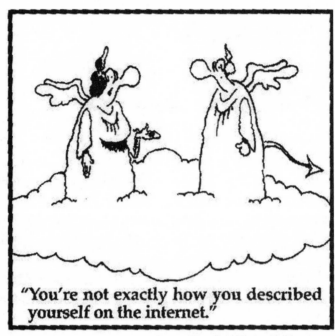

"You're not exactly how you described yourself on the internet."

from *JoyfulNoiseletter.com*
©Scott A. Masear

and Harley L. Schwadron, contributed cartoons to *JN* that were widely reprinted in church publications.

"*JN* editors soon discovered that holy humor, like love, crosses denominational lines, and is an important healing, bridge-building, and peace-making tool. *The editors also discovered that holy humor is the one thing that all the great religions agree on and value unanimously. JN* has attracted subscribers from a variety of faiths that ordinarily rarely communicate.

"The holy fools of *JN* sometimes have gone where angels fear to tread.

"I have read every issue for 30 years. I have all the back issues of *JN* ready for the library of the Gesundheit Institute's Patch Adams Teaching Center and Clinic for Health Professionals we are planning to build in West Virginia."—Patch Adams, MD, *House Calls: How we can all heal the world one visit at a time*

Here is what other people are saying about *The Joyful Noiseletter*:

"*The Joyful Noiseletter* is packed with funny religious stories, plus a page of cartoons, that offer some of the choicest pickings for the pulpit, church bulletins, or dinner table fare." – George W. Cornell, Religion Editor, *The Associated Press*

"Outstanding. This newsletter does what it's supposed to do—it makes you laugh." "Great fun! A joy to read! Useful to church newsletter editors particularly." – *The Associated Church Press*

"Chock-full of digestible tidbits. Highly readable and lots of fun. What a great publication!" – *Evangelical Press Association*

"Here is humor that is reverent and relevant, comical but free of profanity and blasphemy so blatantly featured in the modern media. Impressive graphics and snappy writing fill this newsletter with life and wisdom." –*Catholic Press Association*

"Reading *The Joyful Noiseletter* is like looking at a Norman Rockwell painting. You'll see touches of Americana from glimpses into how we used to be to reminders how we're still the same." –Sandi Dolbee, Religion Editor, *San Diego Union-Tribune*

"JN is a rollicking good idea. We're grateful to its founders for reminding us of humor's rightful place in the life of faith." –*United Methodist Reporter*

"The nondenominational *JN* ministry measures its success not by counting dollars, but by watching people laugh. *JN*'s board of consulting editors includes not only respected Christian leaders, but also an array of denominational representations. JN prints only humor that is tasteful and reverent." –Dan Runyon, *Christianity Today*

"*JN* represents a new generation of clergy, theologians, and comics whose mission is to recapture what they envision as the joyful world of the early Christians, in which the resurrection was a living memory... a movement to a more celebrative faith focusing on joy and fueled by humor." –David Briggs, *The Associated Press*

"It is delightful to note the presence of *JN* in so many congregations across the land. *JN*'s fame is widespread because it easily buries the concept of Christianity as a 'joy-killer.' Truly, it's a 'joy-instiller,' as your witty comments, holy humor, and cartoons bring out in every issue. JN is the best humor publication in Christendom." –Dr. Paul L Maier, best-selling Lutheran author

"What would be my advice to help pastors with their sermons? I would recommend they subscribe to *The Joyful Noiseletter*." –Comedian Steve Allen

"Keep *The Joyful Noiseletter* coming. It's great!" –Joe Garagiola

"What a treasury of HO-HO-Holy Humor! Let us bow our heads and laugh!" –Bil Keane, creator of *The Family Circus*

"*The Joyful Noiseletter* is a gem!" –Johnny Hart, creator of *B.C.*

"It's been such a joy to receive *JN* all these years. You have truly been a 'hand' of God." –Antoinette Bosco, columnist, *Catholic News Service*

"A prominent European theologian once commented that Christianity has no humor. Anyone who thinks this way should subscribe without delay to *The Joyful Noiseletter*." –Sherwood Eliot Wirt, author, *Jesus: Man of Joy*, Billy Graham biographer

"Last year I was given a copy of *JN*, and I really enjoyed it. After I read it, I put it in the men's room at our Quaker church. Thereafter, our Quaker silent worship was punctuated with laughter emanating from the men's room." –Philip Gulley, best-selling Quaker author

"What you have achieved over the past 30 years with that wonderful little publication is nothing short of outstanding. You have touched thousands of lives for the better. Nothing less than having the Holy Spirit bless that ministry—with your talents—could have made it all work. A truly inspiriting legacy." –Lou Jacquet, former editor of *Our Sunday Visitor* and *The Catholic Exponent*, Youngstown, Ohio.

Jokes and Anecdotes

People often use the phrase "deadly serious," but never "deadly humorous." Here are some of our favorite jokes and anecdotes we've published in *The Joyful Noiseletter:*

A man is dying on his deathbed in a Los Angeles hospital. With him are his nurse, his wife, his daughter, and two sons. He knows the end is near so he says to them:

"Sam, I want you to take the Beverly Hills houses." "Sylvia, take the apartments over in Los Angeles Plaza." "Bernie, I want you to take the offices over in City Center." "And Sarah, my dear wife, please take all the residential buildings downtown."

All this boggles the nurse's mind, and as the man slips away, she says to the wife, "Ma'am, your husband must have been such a hardworking man to have accumulated so much property."

The wife replies: "Property shmoperty... the old man had a newspaper route."

Walking home from church, a woman saw a little old man smiling in a rocking chair on a porch. She walked up to him and said, "I couldn't help noticing how happy you look," she said; "What is your secret for a long, happy life?"

"Well, Ma'am," he replied, "I smoke two packs of cigarettes a day, drink seven six-packs of beer a week, eat fatty and greasy fast foods, and never exercise."

"Amazing!" the woman said. "How old are you?"

"Twenty-seven," he said.

A visitor to Israel attended a concert at the Moscovitz Auditorium, and was impressed with the architecture and acoustics. He asked the tour guide, "Is this magnificent auditorium named after Chaim Moscovitz, the famous Talmudic scholar?"

"No," replied the guide. "It is named after Sam Moscovitz, the writer."

"Never heard of him," the visitor said. "What did he write?"

"A check," the guide replied.

At a linguistic conference in London, England, Samsunder Balgobin, a Guyanese, was the clear winner when he answered the following challenging questions:

"Some say there is no difference between 'complete' and 'finished.' Please explain the difference between 'complete' and 'finished' in a way that is easy to understand."

Balgobin rose to the occasion with this answer:

"When you marry the right woman, you are 'complete.' But when you marry the wrong woman, you are 'finished.' And when the right one catches you with the wrong one, you are 'completely finished'!" He got a standing ovation.

A man feared his wife wasn't hearing as well as she used to, and he thought she might need a hearing aid. Not quite sure how to approach her, he called the family doctor to discuss the problem.

The doctor told him there was a simple informal test the husband could perform to give the doctor a better idea about her hearing loss.

"Here's what you do," said the doctor; "stand about 40 feet away from her, and in a normal conversational speaking tone, see if she hears you. If not, go to 30 feet, then 20 feet, and so on, until you get a response."

That evening his wife was in the kitchen cooking dinner. He said to himself, "I'm about 40 feet away; let's see what happens." Then in a normal tone, he asked, "Honey, what's for dinner?" No response.

So the husband moved closer to the kitchen, about 30 feet from his wife and repeated, "Honey, what's for dinner?" Still no response. Next he moved into the dining room, where he was about 20 feet from his wife and asked, "Honey, what's for dinner?" Again no response.

So he walked up to the kitchen door, about 10 feet away: "Honey, what's for dinner?" Again there was no response. So he walked right up behind her: "Honey, what's for dinner?"

"FRED, FOR THE FIFTH TIME, CHICKEN!" she shouted.

A drunk wandered into the back of a church in New York. He stumbled toward an usher, asking, "How long has the pastor been preaching?"

Usher: "About 30 years."

"Well then, I think I'll just stay," said the drunk, adding, "He must be nearly finished."

Signs that your surgeon made a mistake:

His malpractice insurance company was sued for malpractice for insuring him.

When you had a knee replacement, you didn't expect it to be replaced with a hubcap from a 1947 Studebaker roadster.

Every time you went into his office for a follow-up visit, he shouted, "It's alive!"

Your surgeon tells you, "No charge; this one's on me."

In his farewell sermon to his church, the pastor excelled. He was eloquent and well prepared. His text: "In my Father's house are many mansions... I go to prepare a place for you, that where I am there ye may be also." It was later learned that the preacher had accepted a position as chaplain at the local prison.

A paramedic was asked on a local TV talk show program: "What was your most unusual and challenging 911 call?"

"Recently, we got a call from a church," the paramedic said. "A frantic usher said that during the sermon an elderly man passed out in a pew and appeared to be dead. The usher could find no pulse and there was no noticeable breathing."

"What was so unusual and challenging about this particular call?" the interviewer asked.

"Well," the paramedic said, "we carried out four guys before we found the one who was dead."

As a courtesy, a pastor took an elderly church member to the local nursing home to seek information about how they determine whether or not an older person should be put in a nursing home.

"Well," said the nursing home director, "we fill up a bathtub. Then we offer the person a teaspoon, a teacup and a bucket to empty the bathtub."

"Oh, I understand," said the elderly visitor. "A normal person would use the bucket because it's bigger than the spoon or the teacup."

"No," said the administrator, "A normal person would pull the plug. Do you want a bed near a window?"

A middle-aged man went to his doctor for his annual physical. The doctor examined him carefully and ran a battery of tests on him. Finally, he told the man: "I'm sorry to have to tell you this, Mr. Schmidt, but you only have six months to live."

The man left sadly. Six months later he returned to the doctor's office and said, "I'm sorry, doctor, but I can't pay your bill."

So the doctor gave him eight more months.

A kind-hearted English bishop one day observed a woman laboriously pushing a baby buggy up a steep hill. He offered his assistance. When they reached the top of the hill, in answer to her thanks, he said: "Oh, it's nothing at all. I was delighted to do it. As a reward, may I kiss the baby?"

"Baby? Lord bless you sir, it ain't no baby. It's the old man's beer."

A defendant named Joshua stood before a judge in an Amite, Louisiana, courtroom. The judge, who happened to be a Biblical scholar, asked him: "Are you the Joshua who made the sun stand still?"

"No, your honor," the accused man replied, "I'm the Joshua who made the moon shine."

An epitaph on a tombstone read: "Remember, man, as you pass by, as you are now, so once was I. And as I am now, so must you be. Prepare yourself to follow me."

Beneath the epitaph a living wit wrote: "To follow you I'm not content, until I know which way you went."

A doctor, who had a reputation for helping arthritic patients, had a waiting-room full of people. A little old lady, completely bent over in half, shuffled in slowly, leaning on her cane.

When her turn came, she shuffled into the doctor's office, and emerged within half an hour walking completely erect, her head held high. A woman in the waiting room walked up to the little old lady and exclaimed, "It's a miracle! You walked in bent in half and now you're walking erect. What did that doctor do?"

"Miracle, schmiracle," the little old lady replied. "He gave me a longer cane."

Actual questions and answers recorded by a court reporter:

ATTORNEY: "Doctor, before you performed the autopsy, did you check for a pulse?"

DOCTOR: "No."

ATTORNEY: "Did you check for blood pressure?"

DOCTOR: "No"

ATTORNEY: "Did you check for breathing?"

DOCTOR: "No"

ATTORNEY: So, then it is possible that the patient was alive when you began the autopsy?"

DOCTOR: "No"

ATTORNEY: "How can you be so sure, Doctor?"

DOCTOR: "Because his brain was sitting on my desk in a jar."

ATTORNEY: "I see, but could the patient have still been alive, nevertheless?"

DOCTOR: "Yes, it is possible that he could have been alive and practicing law."

A chronic hypochondriac went to his doctor for his annual physical. "Doctor," he said, "Remember those voices I told you I kept hearing in my head? Well, I haven't heard them in a week!"

"That's wonderful news! I'm so happy for you," the doctor exclaimed.

"What's wonderful about it?" the hypochondriac replied. "I'm afraid I'm losing my hearing!"

∾

Worst pieces of advice from a doctor:

"Just sample your Facebook friends and do whatever the consensus opinion on that is."

"You can get the same prescription from a vet for a lot less."

"Take your medications all at once before you leave for vacation so you won't forget to take them while away."

"Eat more and exercise less. I could use the business."

∾

President Ronald Reagan collected Russian jokes. Here's one of Reagan's favorites:

An American and a Russian were talking. The American said, "In America, I can go to the White House, pound on the President's desk, and say, 'I don't like the way you're running the country.'"

The Russian replied, "I can do that! I can go to the Kremlin, walk into Gorbachev's office, pound on his desk, and say, 'I don't like the way President Reagan is running the country.'"

∾

An inexperienced preacher was solemnly conducting his first funeral. Pointing to the body, he declared... "What we have here is only a shell. The nut is already gone."

The HMO Hymn (Sung to the tune of "Old One Hundredth")

Praise God from Whom all blessings flow
That He has moved the HMO.
To reconsider why they pay
After a time of long delay.

Let all that dwell below the skies
Cry out "Unfair!" as we arise.
We never make a payment late,
And yet we must negotiate.

The doctor that we long to see
Has got no time for you and me.
And time with patients he must shirk
To do the endless paperwork.

When Jesus in the manger lay,
So long ago, so far away,
'Twas in a stable, don't you know,
'Cause Mary had an HMO.

Praise God from whom all blessings flow.
And keep us healthy here below.
Send down Your blessings double quick.
We can't afford, Lord, to be sick!

–Brenda W. Quinn, BA,
from *The Journal of Nursing Jocularity*

After telling one of his many jokes to his cabinet, President Lincoln said: "Gentlemen, why do you not laugh? With the fearful strain that is upon me day and night, if I did not laugh, I should die. You need this medicine as much as I do."

The obese G.K. Chesterton once remarked to his lean friend George Bernard Shaw, "To look at you, anyone would think there was a famine in England."

Shaw replied, "To look at you, anyone would think you caused it."

After seeing "Noah," the unbiblical movie extravaganza starring Russell Crowe, a friend of Rev. Karl R. Kraft of Dover, Delaware, reported: "I once had a dream that comedian Jackie Gleason played Noah in the movie. Gleason was spectacular. As the first drops of rain started to fall, Gleason bellowed out, 'And away we go...' Gleason's version, in my dream, seemed to be closer to the Biblical one than Crowe's version."

A well-to-do elderly man in Florida bought a brand-new Corvette and took off with it down a highway. He reached speeds of 90 miles an hour, and soon heard the sirens of a police car chasing him.

The Florida state trooper finally caught up with him and pulled him over. The state trooper said to him, "Sir, I clocked you at 90 miles per hour. Now it's late on Friday and I'd like to get home to my family. I've heard all of the excuses, but if you can tell me one I've never heard before, I'll let you go without a ticket."

The old man replied, "Well, sir, eleven years ago my wife ran off with a Florida state trooper, and I was afraid you were bringing her back."

"Have a good day, sir," said the trooper, motioning him to move on.

The local news station was interviewing an 80-year-old lady because she had just gotten married for the fourth time. The interviewer asked her questions about what it felt like to be marrying again at 80, and then about her new husband's occupation.

"He's a funeral director," she answered.

The newsman then asked her if she wouldn't mind telling him a little about her first three husbands and what they did for a living.

She paused for a few moments, needing time to reflect on all those years. A smile came to her face and she answered proudly, explaining that she had first married a banker when she was in her 20's, then a circus ringmaster when in her 40's, and a preacher when in her 60's, and now—in her 80's—a funeral director.

The interviewer looked at her, quite astonished, and asked why she had married four men with such diverse careers.

"I married one for the money, two for the show, three to get ready, and four to go."

If...

If you can start the day without caffeine,

If you can resist complaining and boring people with your troubles,

If you can eat the same food every day and be grateful for it,

If you can understand when your loved ones are too busy to give you any time,

If you can take criticism and blame without resentment,

If you can conquer tension without medical help,

If you can relax without alcohol,

If you can sleep without the aid of drugs,

Then you are probably the family dog.

This Jewish anecdote will resonate with a lot of Protestants and Catholics as well: During a service at an old synagogue in Eastern Europe, when the Shema prayer was said, half the congregants stood up and half remained sitting.

The half that was seated started yelling at those standing to sit down, and the ones standing, yelled at the ones sitting to stand up.

The rabbi, though learned as he was in the Law and commentaries, didn't know what to do. His congregation suggested that he consult a housebound 98-year-old man who was one of the original founders of their temple.

The rabbi hoped the elderly man would be able to tell him what the actual temple tradition was, so he went to the nursing home with a representative of each faction of the congregation. The one whose followers stood during the Shema said to the old man, "Is it the tradition to stand during this prayer?"

The old man answered, "No, that is not the tradition."

The one whose followers sat, said, "Then it must be the tradition to sit during the Shema!"

The old man answered, "No, that is not the tradition."

Then the rabbi said to the old man, "But the members of the congregation fight all the time, yelling at each other about whether they should sit or stand."

The old man interrupted, exclaiming, "THAT is the tradition."

Do you know how the Prophet Daniel escaped the lions' den after he was thrown into it? He went around to each lion and whispered in his ear: "After dinner there will be speeches."

This true story still makes the rounds and brings chuckles from those who remember the late Rev. Raymond Roden at Trinity Lutheran Church in Webster City, Iowa: After a winter blizzard, Rev. Roden, who was then pastor of Trinity Lutheran, was conducting graveside services in a cemetery where a propane heating device had been used to thaw the ground for the grave opening.

The heater also thawed an area around the grave because as the mourners were being ushered in, a section of the ground gave way and dropped Pastor Roden into the grave under the coffin.

The pastor, covered in mud, came out of the grave clawing at the sides, "However, I completed the graveside service with whatever degree of decorum I was able to muster," he said.

The next day, recounting "the gory details of my recent descent and ascension" to his congregation, Pastor Roden retained his sense of humor. He was leading the liturgy for the Second Sunday of Epiphany and nearly broke up as the Psalm for the day had these lines:

"I waited and waited for the Lord's help, then He listened to me and He heard my cry, and He pulled me out of that dangerous pit; out of a muddy hole."

At a Vatican conference, Pope Francis surprised the cardinals, bishops, and priests by criticizing them for having "funereal faces." The pope said it is a good thing to have a "healthy sense of humor."

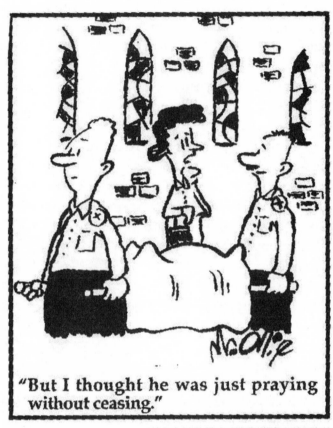

"But I thought he was just praying without ceasing."

from *JoyfulNoiseletter.com*
©Tim Oliphant

Chapter 24

The Doctor Who Avoided Malpractice Suits

A cheerful heart is a good medicine,
but a downcast spirit dries up the bones.

Proverbs 17:22

T hat's the favorite proverb of another *Joyful Noiseletter* consulting editor, Dr. Winslow Fox, 92, a well-known Ann Arbor,
Michigan, family physician.

When Dr. Fox retired, Dr. David K. Fox (no relation), a
spokesman for the Michigan State Medical Society, said, "It's a
remarkable feat to go through a 41-year medical career with just
one minor malpractice suit filed against a physician. Especially in
the state of Michigan, where there's a frenzy in the filing of medical
malpractice suits."

In fact, many of Dr. Fox's patients prayed for him, and Dr. Fox
regularly prayed for them while treating them. Dr. Fox is a longtime advocate of bringing a spiritual dimension to the practice of
medicine, and for many years he was chairman of the Committee on
Medicine and Religion for the Michigan State Medical Association.

Dr. Fox, a long-time member of the First United Methodist
Church of Ann Arbor, would get together with the four physicians
in his office at the start of every week, and pray for their patients.
When he starts his hospital rounds, he will often take a patient's
hand and pray with or for him/her. He says:

> "I believe in spiritual healing. It's usually not an
> instantaneous thing. It's more likely to occur gradually
> over a period of time with a combination of medicine
> and prayer.

"We see people with back disorders who are significantly improved after we pray for them. People with depression or anxiety states also respond favorably to prayer. We've prayed for people with all kinds of conditions."

Dr. Fox is concerned that the medical profession is becoming increasingly secularized. Fox believes the medical profession should be aware that there are gifted healers among the clergy and lay people, and not oppose them. "God works through different instruments," he says.

There is but one temple in this Universe, the Body.

– Thomas Carlyle

According to Dr. Fox, "the way to avoid malpractice suits is to practice good medicine, and to maintain good communications with your patients. It also helps to have patients who are believers and not inclined to sue their physician or anyone else."

Dr. Fox is an avid, lean gardener; and as a Spanish-speaking physician, he has often volunteered his services as a medical missionary to tend to the health needs of poor people, Indians, and Hispanic migrant workers in Arizona, Colorado, and California.

That is his idea of retirement.

Chapter 25

Do We Follow a Depressed Messiah or a Joyful Messiah?

D o we follow a depressed Christ or a joyful Christ? *The Joyful Noiseletter* recently received two dramatically different views on that issue.

We received an email from a Protestant ministry with an article titled, "Did Jesus Battle Depression?" by a young Baptist pastor. The young pastor quoted Isaiah 53:3: "He was despised and rejected, a man of sorrows and acquainted with grief." "Why," he asked, "do we immediately push back the thought that Jesus might have dealt with symptoms of depression? I am of the opinion that Christ did indeed battle depression."

He who gives joy to the world is raised higher among men than he who conquers the world..

–Richard Wagner

This was typical of the super-seriousness of the psychobabble crowd, who for years have been writing articles and books psychoanalyzing Jesus, and suggesting that Jesus was a basket case, a schizophrenic, a manic-depressive, etc., etc.

About the same time, Bill Reynolds of Paltaka, Florida, sent us a commentary by Catherine Marshall, the wife of U.S. Senate Chaplain Peter Marshall. Catherine Marshall saw Jesus as a man of joy and good humor.

Some years ago, Catherine Marshall wrote: "Many preachers have emphasized Christ as 'the man of sorrows' but have almost completely ignored the fact that Jesus loved people, loved to mingle with them, loved to laugh and to engage in light banter with them, and had a rare sense of humor."

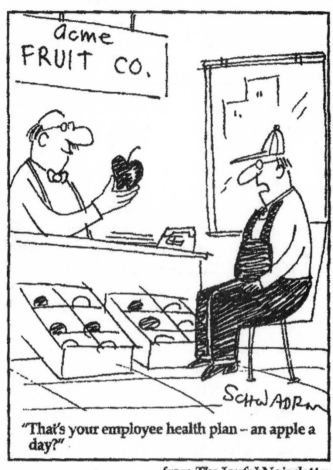

"That's your employee health plan -- an apple a day?"

from *The Joyful Noiseletter*
©Harley L. Schwadron

When she was bedridden and despondent for several years with a serious lung ailment, she suddenly awoke one night in total darkness, and sensed a powerful Presence in her room.

"Why do you take yourself so seriously?" the Presence asked her. "Relax! There's nothing I can't take care of."

The Presence was loving and almost merry, with a teasing, light banter. The encounter was a turning point in her illness and put her on the road to good health.

"The Jesus I had met was oh, so different from the Jesus pictured in most Sunday school books or painted by most artists—solemn, sad-eyed, plodding on His sorrowful way to Calvary."

Later, Marshall was delighted when the Quaker theologian Dr. Elton Trueblood authored a book titled, *The Humor of Christ.*

"One obvious reason why we have not recognized so much of Jesus' humor: we are missing the tone of voice and the facial expression," Marshall wrote. "This is a great loss, for much of a person's wit and banter are revealed by his happy expression and personality."

Joy, like worship itself, is revolutionary, liberating, dangerous, and counter-cultural, enabling us to resist the forces that would seek to enslave us, and to laugh at their absurdities.

–Richard Johnson in his commentary on *Acts*

The New Testament is full of Scriptures attesting to the appearance of a joyful Messiah. Who but the Messiah could talk about joy to his disciples before he knew he was about to be whipped, scourged, humiliated, and crucified?

While Jesus sometimes experienced grief, and wept on occasion, he was far from a depressive. He was a joyful Spirit when he walked on this earth, and even more joyful when he ascended to heaven. Children and the sick were attracted to Jesus. Children and the sick are not attracted to depressives. No depressive would have urged his followers to "be of good cheer."

Martin Luther said, "If you want to define Christ rightly, then pay heed to how the angel defines him, namely 'a great joy,'" Luther added: "Flee from sorrow and serve God with joy... If you're not allowed to laugh in heaven, I don't want to go there."

In his *Table Talks*, Luther reported that on the first day of Christmas, 1538, he was overcome by feelings of great joy. He exclaimed:

> "Oh, we wretched people! To think that we are so cold and unresponsive to this great joy given to us, this great benefaction, which is far, far superior to all other works of creation, and is nevertheless met with such weak faith, which was preached to us by angels, who were heavenly theologians and who were so joyful on our behalf!"

The English Baptist preacher Charles Spurgeon (1834–1892), who admitted he occasionally suffered from depression, said: "In your most depressed seasons, you are to get joy and peace through believing in Christ."

Many other religious figures down through the centuries, including St. Francis of Assisi and John Wesley, saw Christ as a God of joy.

Do you follow a depressed Messiah or a joyful Messiah?

Chapter 26

Healing Prayers for Hard Times

In one of her delightful books, *At Wit's End*, humorist Erma Bombeck tells this story:

> "In church the other Sunday, I was intent on a small child who was turning around smiling at everyone. He wasn't gurgling, spitting, humming, kicking, tearing the hymnals, or rummaging through his mother's handbag. He was just smiling.
>
> "Finally, his mother jerked him about and in a stage whisper that could be heard in a little theater off-Broadway said: 'Stop that grinning! You're in church!' With that, she gave him a belt and as the tears rolled down his cheeks, added, 'That's better,' and returned to her prayers.
>
> "We sing, 'Make a joyful noise unto the Lord!' while our faces reflect the sadness of one who has just buried a rich aunt who left everything to her pregnant hamster.
>
> "Suddenly I was angry. It occurred to me the entire world is in tears, and if you're not, then you'd better get with it. I wanted to grab this child with the tear-stained face close to me and tell him about my God. The happy God. The smiling God. The God who had to have a sense of humor to have created the likes of us.
>
> "I wanted to tell him He is an understanding God. One who understands little children who pick their noses in church because they are bored. I wanted to tell him I've taken a few lumps in my time for daring to smile at religion. By tradition, one wears faith with the solemnity

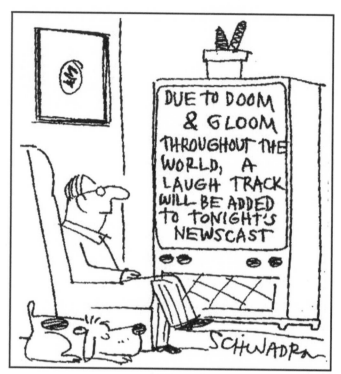

from *JoyfulNoiseletter.com*
©Harley L. Schwadron

of a mourner, the gravity mask of tragedy, and the dedication o a Rotary badge.

"What a fool, I thought. Here was a woman sitting next to the only thing left in our civilization—the only hope, our miracle—our only promise of infinity. If he couldn't smile in church, where was there left to go?"

The famous peace prayer of St. Francis is also a healing prayer:

Lord, make me an instrument of Thy peace.
Where there is hatred, let me sow love;
Where there is injury, pardon;
Where there is doubt, faith;
Where there is despair, hope;
Where there is darkness, light;
Where there is sadness, joy.
O Master, grant that I may not so much seek
To be consoled as to console;
To be understood as to understand;
To be loved as to love;
For it is in giving that we receive;
It is in pardoning that we are pardoned;
And it is in dying that we are born to eternal life.

When Rev. Dr. Karl R. Kraft of Dover, Delaware, read Dick Van Dyke's memoir, *My Life in and Out of Show Business* (Crown/Archetype, NY), he was delighted to discover this prayer by an unknown author that Van Dyke gave at the funeral of his longtime friend Stan Laurel:

God bless all clowns
Who star in the world with laughter,
Who ring the rafters with flying jest,
Who make the world spin merry on its way.

God bless all the clowns.
So poor the world would be,
Lacking their piquant touch, hilarity,
The belly laughs, the ringing lovely.

God bless all the clowns.
Give them a long, good life,
Make bright their way—they're a race apart.
Alchemists most, who turn their hearts' pain
Into a dazzling jest to lift the heart.

God bless all clowns.

The Clown's Prayer

As I stumble through this life,
Help me to create more laughter than tears,
Dispense more happiness than gloom,
Spread more cheer than despair.

Never let me become so indifferent
That I fail to see he wonder
In the eyes of the child
Or the twinkle in the eyes of the aged.

Never let me forget that my total effort
Is to cheer people, make them happy
And forget at least momentarily
All the unpleasantness in their lives.

And in my final moment,
May I hear you whisper,
When you made my people smile,
You made me smile.

          –Author Unknown

I start every morning with this prayer:

Dear Lord: Restore the joy of my salvation, my sense of humor, and my physical fitness so that I can better serve You and others.

And never forget the famous commencement address of Winston Churchill after World War II. Churchill got up and told the graduates: "Never, never, never, never, never, never, never, never, never, never, never, never give up."

He then sat down to a thunderous ovation.

When things go wrong
As they sometimes will,
When the road you're trudging
Seems all up hill,
When the funds are low
And the debts are high,
And you want to smile,
But you have to sigh,
When care is pressing you down a bit
Rest, if you must, but don't you quit.

–Author unknown

We all have to realize that our health is the most important thing in our lives, and we all must do everything we can to preserve it. Prevention is also a life issue.

I've known sickly millionaires who would have given their entire fortune for one week of good health.

What does it profit a person to gain the whole world and lose their health?

It has sometimes been said that churches are "hospitals for the sick." If that is so, isn't it the responsibility of churches to teach people how to live a healthy lifestyle?

"It is really a natural trend to lapse into taking oneself too seriously because it's the easiest thing to do, for solemnity and seriousness flow out of us naturally, but laughter is a leap into light. It is easy to be heavy, hard to be light. And never forget that Satan fell by force of gravity."

–G.K. Chesterton

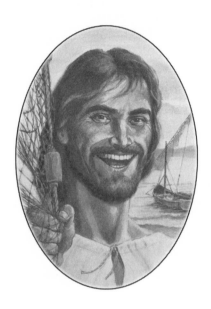

Recommended Reading

Books on Healthful Living

The Blue Zones: Lessons for Living Longer from the People Who've Lived the Longest by Dan Buettner (National Geographic Society)

Primitive Physick by John Wesley (Amazon.com)

Dr. John Harvey Kellogg and the Religion of Biologic Living by Prof. Brian C. Wilson (Indiana University Press)

Healthful Living by Ellen White (Adventist Book Center, Amazon.com)

The Ministry of Healing by Ellen White (Adventist Books, Amazon.com)

House Calls: How We Can All Heal the World one Visit at a Time by Patch Adams, M.D. (Robert D. Reed Publishers)

Gesundheit! Patch Adams, M.D. (Healing Arts Press)

God, Health, and Happiness by Scott Morris, M.D. (Barbour Press, Church Health Center)

The Holy Unmercenary Doctors and Healers of the Orthodox Church (Translated from the Greek) by Georgia Hronas (Light and Life Publishing)

What the Bible Says about Healthy Living by Rex Russell, M.D. (Regal Books)

Why Christians Get Sick by Rev. Dr. George H. Malkmus (Destiny Image Publishers)

Sugar Blues by William Duffy (Amazon.com)

Nature's Best Remedies: The World of Health and Healing All Around You (National Geographic Society)

The Food and Feasts of Jesus: The Original Mediterranean Diet, with Menus and Recipes by Douglas Neel and Joel Pugh (Rowman and Littlefield)

100 Simple Things You Can Do to Prevent Alzheimer's by Jean Carper (Little Brown and Company)

J'Arming by Dale L. Anderson, M.D. (Amazon.com)

My First 100 Years: A Look Back from the Finish Line by Waldo McBurney (Leathers Publishing)

Hoffer's Laws of Natural Nutrition by Dr. Abram Hoffer, M.D. (Quarry Press, Ontario)

Supersize Me by Morgan Spurlock (Lennex Corp., Scotland)

Books on the Healing Power of Humor

The Joyful Christ: The Healing Power of Humor by Cal Samra (HarperCollins, Amazon.com)

The Humor of Christ by Elton Trueblood (HarperCollins, Amazon.com)

The Sacred Art of Clowning... and Life! by Cleone Lyvonne Reed (Robert D. Reed Publishers)

Jesus: Man of Joy by Sherwood Eliot Wirt (Harvest House)

Laughter Was God's Idea: Stories about Healing Humor by Chaplain Jack Hinson (joyfulnoiseletter.com)

This Won't Hurt a Bit! and Other Fractured Truths in Health Care by Karen Buxman, RN (karenbuxman.com)

Joyfully Aging by Dr. Richard Bimler (Concordia Publishing House)

Laughter Is the Best Medicine by Dave Coverly (Sellers Publishing)

Holy Humor by Cal and Rose Samra (Guideposts Books, joyfulnoiseletter.com)

More Holy Humor by Cal and Rose Samra (Guideposts Books, joyfulnoiseletter.com)

More Holy Hilarity by Cal and Rose Samra (Guideposts Books, joyfulnoiseletter.com)

Do Vegetarians Eat Animal Crackers? by Robert Bimler (joyfulnoiseletter.com)

Just Play Ball by Joe Garagiola (National Book Network, joyfulnoiseletter.com)

The Funny Side of Tennis by Cal Samra with Bil Keane, Charles M. Schulz, and 9 other cartoonists. joyfulnoiseletter.com)

Recommended Viewing

Supersize Me (DVD) Morgan Spurlock (Amazon.com)

Food, Inc. (DVD) Eric Schlosser, Robert Kenner (Amazon.com)

Fed Up (DVD) Stephanie Soeghtig and Katie Couric (Amazon.com)

That Sugar Film (DVD) Damon Gameau (Amazon.com)

About the Author

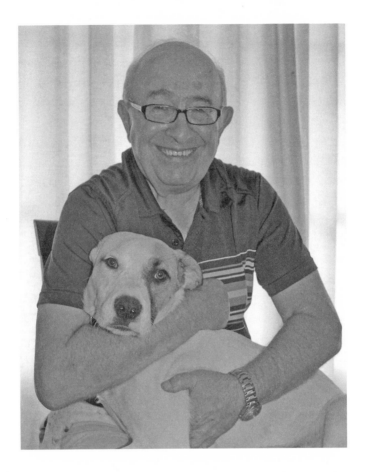

Cal Samra is the founding editor and publisher of *The Joyful Noiseletter*, a national humor newsletter that for thirty years has provided jokes that pastors can tell and reproducible cartoons for church editors of all faith traditions. *The Joyful Noiseletter* has received awards of excellence from The Associated Church Press, The Catholic Press Association, and the Evangelical Press Association. Lutheran author and Pastor Paul L. Maier called *The Joyful Noiseletter* the best humor publication in Christendom.

Prior to his debut as a humorist, Samra had extensive experience as a newspaper journalist. He was editorial direction of *The Michigan Daily* at the University of Michigan, a reporter and columnist for *The Ann Arbor News*, a reporter for the Associated press' Detroit Bureau, a reporter for *The Flint Journal*, a reporter and columnist for *The Battle Creek Enquirer*, a copyreader for *The New York Herald Tribune*, and a reporter for *The Newark Evening News* in New Jersey.

In the 1960s, Samra served as the lay executive director and newsletter editor of what became the Huxley Institute for Biosocial Research, named in honor of Sir Julian Huxley and his brother, Aldous Huxley. The institute had a distinguished board of psychiatric researchers exploring the physiology, biochemistry, and nutritional factors in severe mental illnesses.

Samra is the author of a dozen humor books. His book, *The Joyful Christ: The Healing Power of Humor*, published by HarperCollins in 1985, launched *The Joyful Noiseletter* after many pastors and church editors requested a newsletter that would provide them with clean humor and cartoons on a regular basis.

His books, *Holy Humor, More Holy Humor, Holy Hilarity,* and *More Holy Hilarity*, published by Guideposts, Thomas Nelson, and Waterbrook Press have sold a million copies.

Not only has Samra's professional life led him to writing this book full of wisdom, but also his personal life. After a serious illness, the author himself recovered his health when he returned to the natural Mediterranean diet he had been raised on—very similar to the food that Jesus ate.

Samra's keen interest has always been physical fitness, organic gardening, and nutrition. Next to his Christian faith and family, tennis is his great love. One of the favorite books he wrote is *The Funny Side of Tennis*, full of tennis humor and cartoons published by *The Joyful Noiseletter*. At age 85, this court jester still plays tennis with his aging but young-at-heart friends four times a week.

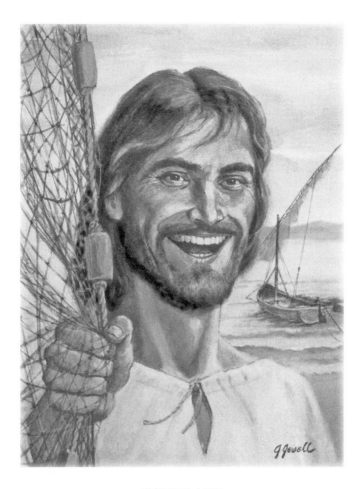

COVER ART

"The Risen Christ by the Sea" by Jack Jewell.
Copyright © by The Joyful Noiseletter.

Full-color framed and unframed prints in various sizes may be ordered from www.joyfulnoiseletter.com or by calling toll-free 1-800-877-2757.

ROBERT D. REED PUBLISHERS ORDER FORM

Call in your order for fast service and quantity discounts.
(541) 347-9882

Or order online at www.rdrpublishers.com *using Paypal.*
OR order by mail: Make a copy of this form; enclose payment information:
Robert D. Reed Publishers, P.O. Box 1992, Bandon, OR 97411
Fax: (541) 347-9883

Send indicated books to:

Name _____

Address _____

City _____ State _____ Zip _____

Phone _____ Cell _____

E-mail _____

Payment by check ___ or credit card ___ *(All major credit cards accepted.)*

Name on card _____

Card Number _____

Exp. Date _____ 3-digit number on back of card _____

Quantity		**Total**
_____ *The Physically Fit Messiah* (Cal Samra)	$14.95	_____
_____ *House Calls* (Patch Adams, MD)	$11.95	_____
_____ *The Sacred Art of Clowning (Cleone Reed)*	$14.95	_____
_____ *The Kid's Herb Book* (Lesley Tiarra)	$19.95	_____
_____ *Let's Eat* (Dr. J. Renae Norton)	$17.95	_____
_____ *How Maji Gets Mongo off the Couch* (Dr. Norton)	$17.95	_____
_____ *Remembering Pets* (Gina Dalpra-Berman)	$14.95	_____
_____ Other books from website: _____		

Total Number of Books _____ Total Amount _____

Note: Shipping is $4.50 1st book + $1 for each additional book.
FREE Shipping on orders over $25.00

Shipping _____

THE TOTAL _____

Thank you for your order.